Baillière's

CLINICAL
INFECTIOUS
DISEASES

INTERNATIONAL PRACTICE AND RESEARCH

Baillière's

CLINICAL INFECTIOUS DISEASES

INTERNATIONAL PRACTICE AND RESEARCH

Volume 2/Number 2
July 1995

Malaria

G. PASVOL MA, MBChB, DPhil, FRCP
Guest Editor

Baillière Tindall
London Philadelphia Sydney Tokyo Toronto

This book is printed on acid-free paper.

Baillière Tindall 24–28 Oval Road,
W. B. Saunders   London NW1 7DX, UK
Company Ltd
                 The Curtis Center, Independence Square West,
                 Philadelphia, PA 19106–3399, USA

                 55 Horner Avenue
                 Toronto, Ontario M8Z 4X6, Canada

                 Harcourt Brace & Company
                 Australia
                 30–52 Smidmore Street, Marrickville, NSW 2204, Australia

                 Harcourt Brace & Company
                 Japan Inc,
                 Ichibancho Central Building, 22-1
                 Ichibancho, Chiyoda-ku, Tokyo 102, Japan

ISSN 1071–6564

ISBN 0–7020–1983–6 (single copy)

Baillière's Clinical Infectious Diseases is published three times each year by Baillière Tindall. Prices for Volume 2 (1995) are:

TERRITORY	ANNUAL SUBSCRIPTION	SINGLE ISSUE
Europe including UK	£78.00 (Institutional) post free	£30.00 post free
	£58.00 (Individual) post free	
All other countries	Consult your local Harcourt Brace & Company office	

The editor of this publication is Ian Bramley, Baillière Tindall,
24–28 Oval Road, London NW1 7DX.

Baillière's Clinical Infectious Diseases is covered in Current Contents/Clinical Medicine, the Science Citation Index, SciSearch, and Research Alert.

Typeset by Phoenix Photosetting, Chatham.
Printed and bound in Great Britain by the University Printing House, Cambridge.

Contributors to this issue

ROBERTO AMADOR MD, Assistant Professor, Instituto de Inmunologia, Hospital San Juan de Dios, Universidad Nacional Colombia, AA 44709, Bogota, Colombia.

DAVID J. BRADLEY MA, DM, FRCP, FRCPath, FFPHM, FIBiol, HonFIWEM, Co-Director of PHLS Malaria Reference Library; Consultant in Public Health Medicine, North Thames RHA; Professor of Tropical Hygiene, London School of Hygiene and Tropical Medicine, University of London, Keppel Street, London, WC1E 7HT, UK.

JAN CARLSSON PhD, Research Assistant, St Mary's Hospital Medical School, Imperial College of Science, Technology and Medicine, Lister Unit, Northwick Park Hospital, Harrow, Middlesex HA1 3UJ, UK.

BARBARA CLOUGH PhD, Research Assistant, St Mary's Hospital Medical School, Imperial College of Science, Technology and Medicine, Lister Unit, Northwick Park Hospital, Harrow, Middlesex HA1 3UK, UK.

ROSS L. COPPEL MBBS, DTM&H, PhD, Professor, Department of Microbiology, Monash University, Clayton, Melbourne, Victoria 3168, Australia.

MAY HO BSc, MSc, MD, FRCP(C), Associate Professor, Department of Microbiology and Infectious Diseases, University of Calgary, 3330 Hospital Drive NW, Calgary, Alberta, T2N 4N1, Canada.

DOMINIC KWIATKOWSKI MRCP, Medical Research Council Senior Clinical Fellow and Honorary Consultant, Department of Paediatrics, John Radcliffe Hospital, Headington, Oxford, OX3 9DU, UK.

MALCOLM E. MOLYNEUX MB, BChir, MS, FRCP, Honorary Consultant Physician, Mersey Region; Professor of Tropical Medicine, Liverpool School of Tropical Medicine, Pembroke Place, Liverpool, L3 5QA, UK.

ALBERTO MORENO MD, Researcher, Instituto de Inmunologia, Hospital San Juan de Dios, Universidad Nacional de Colombia, AA 44709, Bogota, Colombia.

GEOFFREY PASVOL MA, MBChB, DPhil, FRCP, Professor in Infection and Tropical Medicine, St Mary's Hospital Medical School, Imperial College of Science, Technology and Medicine, Lister Unit, Northwick Park Hospital, Harrow, Middlesex HA1 3UJ, UK.

MANUEL E. PATARROYO MD, Director, Instituto de Inmunologia, Hospital San Juan de Dios, Universidad Nacional de Colombia, AA 44709, Bogota, Colombia.

MARIO ALBERTO POSADA BSc, MSc, Researcher, Instituto de Inmunologia, Hospital San Juan de Dios, Universidad Nacional de Colombia, AA 44709, Bogota, Colombia.

MAURICIO ROJAS MD, Researcher, Instituto de Inmunologia, Hospital San Juan de Dios, Universidad Nacional de Colombia, AA 44709, Bogota, Colombia.

MARY M. SEXTON BSc, PhD, Research Associate, Department of Microbiology and Infectious Diseases, University of Calgary, 3330 Hospital Drive NW, Calgary, Alberta T2N 4N1, Canada.

G. DENNIS SHANKS MD, MPH, LtCol, Deputy Commander, US Army Medical Research Unit—Kenya, Unit 64109, Box 401, APO AE 09831-4109, USA.

GEORGES SNOUNOU PhD, Research Fellow, St Mary's Hospital Medical School, Imperial College of Science, Technology and Medicine, Lister Unit, Northwick Park Hospital, Harrow, Middlesex HA1 3UJ, UK.

NICHOLAS J. WHITE DSc, MD, FRCP, Director, Wellcome–Mahidol University Oxford Tropical Medicine Research Programme, Faculty of Tropical Medicine, Mahidol University, 420/6 Rajvithi Road, Bangkok, 10400, Thailand.

PETER A. WINSTANLEY MD, MRCP, DTM&H, Senior Lecturer, Department of Pharmacology and Therapeutics, University of Liverpool, Liverpool L69 3BX; Consultant Physician, Royal Liverpool University Hospital, Liverpool, L7 8XP, UK.

Table of contents

PREVIOUS ISSUES

Vol 1, No. 1 1994
Cytokines in Infection
G. E. Griffin

Vol. 1, No. 2 1994
Strategies for Intracellular Survival of Microbes
D. G. Russell

Vol. 1, No. 3 1994
Infections in Immunocompromised Oncological Patients
M. P. Glauser & T. Calandra

Vol. 2, No. 1 1995
Invasive Fungal Infections in Cancer Patients
F. Meunier

FORTHCOMING ISSUE

Vol. 2, No. 3 1995
Pneumocystis carinii
F. R. Sattler & P. D. Walzer

Preface

Ever since the identification of the aetiological agent of malaria, by Charles Louis Alphonse Laveran in 1880, advances in malaria have paralleled those of modern medical science. The presence of the subject of malaria at the moving edge of modern medicine has been particularly true in the last two decades, with the recent advances of molecular, cellular and immunological methods. In this respect malaria can hold its head high; the subject has captivated an increasing cadre of talented and enthusiastic scientists, basic and clinical, who have been fascinated by one of the most sophisticated and complex infections of man. The last book dealing in its entirety with clinical aspects of malaria was published in 1986, but since then the field has evolved rapidly.

It is hoped that this up-to-date volume will be of particular interest to clinicians who have the curiosity and the desire to learn more about the background science of malaria, and perhaps those scientists who would like to increase their clinical perspective of the disease. In this volume I have tried to bring together those world experts who have had extensive practical experience of malaria in a wide variety of clinical settings. Malaria is a clinical subject which has something of interest for most, and the emerging picture is one where the disease differs widely from one geographical and population setting to the next.

Whilst the major aim of this volume is to provide information on clinical understanding and management, it is hoped that it will also answer the many questions that clinicians have with regard to some of the more fascinating areas of subject, as well as raising some of the controversies and other areas which remain unresolved.

My task was made that much simpler because of the enthusiastic response by my malarialogical colleagues throughout the world and I must thank them for their very prompt efforts and attention to detail which has allowed this volume to appear so rapidly. I certainly hope that this book will bring more enthusiasts and talent to bear on this important infection which continues to afflict so much of humanity.

G. PASVOL

1

The epidemiology of malaria in the tropics and in travellers

DAVID J. BRADLEY

It is true of malaria, more than any other infection, that the clinician who does not understand the epidemiology of the disease cannot properly understand, manage, or advise his or her patients. The epidemiology of malaria is unusually diverse, so much so that two clinicians, one practising in Sri Lanka and the other in Ghana or Nigeria, might believe they were dealing with different diseases, were it not for the evidence under the microscope. For the Sri Lankan, malaria is an epidemic disease of great unpredictability, affecting all ages and with the disruptive power of a big influenza epidemic in Europe but a higher mortality, affecting whole families and villages for several weeks before abating and then lying low for several years. By contrast, the West African physician has never seen a malaria epidemic: everyone becomes infected from a few weeks of age onwards, and at any time over three quarters of the primary school children will have parasites in their blood. It is an illness of early childhood and of infancy and in the absence of prompt medical care may kill 5–10% of all children born, while adults are much less troubled by the disease unless they travel to other areas. This chapter aims to explain these differences in indigenous malaria and also the epidemiology of risk to travellers from temperate countries who visit endemic areas.

BASIC EPIDEMIOLOGY OF THE PARASITES

The basic epidemiology of human malaria has been known for almost a century (Ross, 1910). Malaria parasites are either within people or in the bodies of female anopheline mosquitoes. There is, for practical purposes, no animal reservoir and no free-living stage of the parasites. The life cycle is therefore a two-phase cycle (Figure 1). Variation in the stages in the mosquito vector, traditionally known as the 'extrinsic cycle', is responsible for the main epidemiological differences between places, while aspects of the human population provide upper limits to malaria transmission and disease. Non-immune travellers who are foolish enough to ignore prophylactic measures provide an indication of levels of transmission and risk, rather as the canaries that used to be taken down the mines

Baillière's Clinical Infectious Diseases—
Vol. 2, No. 2, July 1995
ISBN 0–7020–1983–6

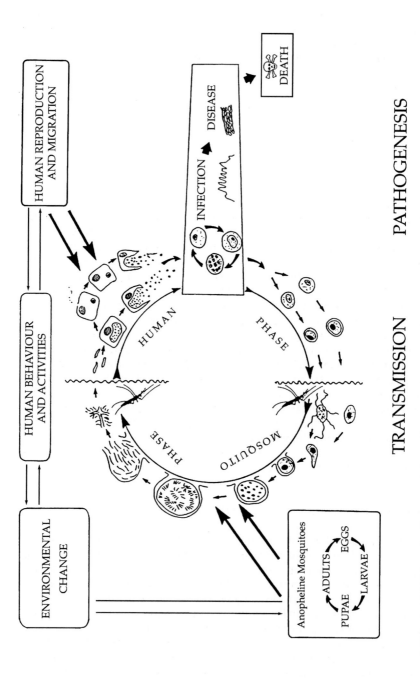

Figure 1. Diagram of the life cycle of human malaria parasites, also including some factors affecting transmission. From Targett (1991, *Malaria, Waiting for the Vaccine.* Chichester: Wiley) with permission.

provided an indication of air quality. Those who practice medicine in temperate countries need to keep a sense of proportion: imported malaria comprises less than 1 in 10 000 of malaria cases in the world.

Malaria is one of the main causes of infant and young child mortality in sub-Saharan Africa, where health records are least complete, so that estimates of global malaria mortality are in the range of 1–2 million or even more, and estimated morbidity is given by WHO as 170 million annually, probably a low estimate. The global point prevalence of parasitaemia is surely much higher.

There are four species of human malaria parasite. Of these, *Plasmodium falciparum* is clinically the most important because its schizonts, or dividing stages in the red cells, cause the erythrocytes to become sticky and adherent to the capillary endothelium of deep organs so that there is sludging of the cerebral blood flow and in non-immunes a substantial risk of cerebral anoxia, coma and progression to death: cerebral malaria. The sporozoites, or infective stages in the mosquito salivary glands, are inoculated by mosquito bite into the bloodstream, where they pass rapidly to the liver and penetrate parenchymal cells within a few hours. In the case of *P. falciparum* they develop there for 5 days and then merozoites burst out having multiplied 30 000-fold, and penetrate the red cells where they undergo a 48-hour cycle of replication which continues until ended by death of the patient or regulated by host responses (Garnham, 1988). All the liver stages from a cohort of sporozoites develop at once so there are no late relapses. In travellers who have returned to an area free of malaria transmission, over 98% of cases will have become manifest within 3 months. Treatment that clears the bloodstream of parasites effects a radical cure. Falciparum malaria due to a single mosquito bite and left untreated, if the victim survives, will keep the patient parasitaemic for 3–6 months. During perhaps two thirds of this time there will be forms infective to mosquitoes (gametocytes, also called crescents in the case of *P. falciparum*, because of their shape) circulating in the blood.

The mildest of the human malarias, *P. malariae*, resembles *P. falciparum* in lacking persistent forms in the liver, but the proliferation cycle in the red cells is 72 hours. Parasitaemias tend to be low and are easily missed, especially in mixed infections. However, the blood stages may persist for many years in the absence of chemotherapy (Garnham, 1977).

Plasmodium vivax can complete its extrinsic cycle in the mosquito at lower temperatures than *P. falciparum* and therefore has a wider distribution. It has been transmitted in the UK and the Netherlands within the last century. At a given temperature its extrinsic cycle will be shorter than that of *P. falciparum* and consequently it can spread more rapidly through a non-immune community. In a malaria epidemic, therefore, vivax cases will predominate in the early stages of the outbreak, and falciparum cases will preponderate in the later stages (Macdonald, 1957). Exoerythrocytic vivax parasites tend to persist in the liver parenchymal cells as hypnozoites and may give rise to late relapses, even after several years (Krotoski et al, 1982). Some *P. vivax* strains from areas such as Romania with a very short transmission season (such that it will be over before parasites contracted at the beginning can complete a transmission cycle) give rise entirely to hypnozoites and create a prolonged incubation and pre-patent period of almost a year's duration (Garnham et al, 1975). *Plasmodium ovale* resembles *P. vivax* in its biology and effectively replaces vivax in West Africa where the indigenous population has Duffy blood group negative red cells which are resistant to *P. vivax* infection (Miller et al, 1976).

EPIDEMIOLOGY AS DETERMINED BY THE VECTORS

Mosquitoes fall into two broad categories: the culicines which are more numerous in species but are not susceptible to the malaria parasites of man, and the anophelines, most species of which are susceptible to the human malaria parasite strains found in their local vicinity. Only the female feeds on blood and can therefore be a malaria vector. A blood feed is needed for maturation of the eggs of the mosquito so that the life of an adult female mosquito is a series of cycles of feeding on blood, resting to allow the meal to digest and eggs to mature, flight to a potential breeding place to lay eggs and renewed search for a blood feed. This feeding cycle can be as short as 2 days, though it is often longer. If the feed is on someone with circulating malaria parasite gametocytes, the anopheline may become infected and gametes are released in the mosquito gut, fuse, migrate to the stomach wall and develop. Eventually this stage, the oocyst, ruptures and multiple infective forms migrate to the salivary glands to render the mosquito infective to people for the rest of her life. From infection to first becoming infectious to people takes around 10–12 days in the tropics, the duration of the extrinsic cycle. This is prolonged at lower temperatures and is not completed at temperatures below 15°C for *P. vivax*, warmer for *P. falciparum* (Macdonald, 1952; Figure 2).

Although the biology and ecology of anopheline mosquitoes is complex and known in great detail, there are only five variable aspects of mosquito life that directly affect malaria transmission and these can be reduced to three for most purposes, as anophelines can usually be assumed to be susceptible to the local malaria and two aspects of feeding behaviour can be combined. The three key variables then become mosquito density, feeding and longevity. It is clear that the more mosquitoes the greater the degree of malaria transmission, because there will be more mosquitoes to pick up malaria from each person with gametocytes and to pass it on. The relationship is linear; transmission potential is proportional to mosquito density. There are two aspects of mosquito feeding behaviour: the frequency of feeding, which can be as high as 0.5/night with a 2 day cycle, and the choice of host. Since human malaria is effectively species-specific a mosquito feed on domestic stock or birds can be ignored so far as malaria transmission is concerned (however much the meal matters to the mosquito), and the feeding frequency can be multiplied by the probability that the feed is on human beings to give a measure of the man-biting habit. This can have a value up to 0.5 for the highly efficient African malaria vectors of the *Anopheles gambiae* complex or low, for example, 0.07 for a

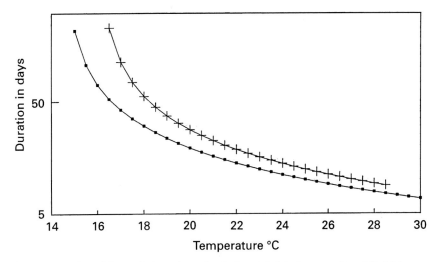

Figure 2. Duration of the extrinsic cycle, or incubation period in the mosquito, of *P. falciparum* (—+—) and *P. vivax* (—■—) in relation to ambient temperature.

mosquito that feeds every third night and only selects people as its victims 20% of the time (0.33×0.2). Moreover, because the mosquito has to feed on people at least twice to transmit malaria, once to catch the infection and once to pass it on, transmission is proportional to the square of the man-biting habit. Longevity is even more crucial, since a mosquito has got to survive for at least the duration of the extrinsic cycle, over 10 days, after catching malaria if it is to pass on the infection, and 10 days is quite a long time in the life of a female mosquito which may have a daily mortality of 5–25% (Macdonald, 1952).

It follows that a long-lived anopheline that feeds frequently and preferentially on people, *An. gambiae* (complex) and *An. funestus* in Africa, *An. minimus* in western Asia, will transmit malaria much more effectively than a zoophilic species that prefers other animals, feeds less frequently and is short-lived, such as *An. culicifacies* in India or Sri Lanka or *An. superpictus* in Africa. Transmission may be measured by the basic case reproduction rate (BCRR), the average number of cases to which one malaria case would give rise, before recovering or dying, after a single generation of passage through mosquitoes and assuming that the surrounding people are non-immunes. The BCRR may be 100 or even 1000 times greater for the long-lived man-biting mosquitoes than the others, and the pattern of malaria resulting is known as stable or unstable malaria, respectively.

The most stable malaria is found in Africa, especially rural West and East Africa where the BCRR of up to 1000 means that there is a 1000-fold more transmission than is needed to keep the parasites in being. Consequently everyone is infected in infancy or very soon after. People may be subjected to several infective bites each night and superinfections are the rule; clinical disease preponderates amongst the very young who suffer severe anaemia in infancy and also cerebral malaria shortly after.

Immunity is gradually acquired under this onslaught of parasites: this first reduces the frequency of disease and the numbers of infective gametocytes, then lowers the levels of the erythrocytic stages and only by adolescence does it lead to the absence of circulating parasites from the majority of the population (Davidson, 1955). For much of childhood most of the inhabitants have a parasitaemia, whether they are well or febrile, and much ingenuity has been expended in attempting to define when a fever is due to malaria and when it is simply concomitant with the parasitaemia but due to other infective causes. There is no absolute answer to this question in an individual case.

Because of the intensity of transmission, those who reach adult life in areas of stable (or holoendemic) malaria have substantial immunity to many strains of the predominant *P. falciparum* malaria, will be subject to occasional parasitaemia and fever, getting much iller during the first pregnancy when immunity appears to fall (Brabin, 1983), and also becoming febrile after travel to other endemic (and possibly also non-endemic) areas.

Attempts at control of stable malaria have been relatively unsuccessful and have not been attempted over much of sub-Saharan Africa. To stop transmission would require up to a 1000-fold reduction, which is beyond the technical means available, even if meticulously and expensively implemented. This very high level of endemicity creates a substantial risk for the traveller from a temperate country who visits there, and attack rates of 2% are reached among short-term visitors from the UK to West Africa (Phillips-Howard et al, 1990).

Unstable malaria, as found in Sri Lanka, North West India, and many other areas occurs where the short-lived zoophilic anopheline vectors achieve a BCRR of just over 1, the level below which malaria is unable to sustain itself. Because the determinants of malaria will not be steady but vary due to weather and other environmental changes, the BCRR will occasionally rise well above 1, for example if unusual monsoon rains suddenly increase breeding sites for *An. culicifacies*. A BCRR rise to 10 will mean that 1 case gives rise to 10, those 10 lead to 100, the 100 produce 1000, and it is easy to see how an epidemic develops. Such epidemics reach the headlines because of the disruptive effects of sudden illness affecting most of the population, but chances of control in these circumstances are good since the BCRR is not very far above 1 and it is feasible to reduce it by practical control measures. The level of transmission is much lower than in stable malaria and, except at the very height of the epidemic, the hazard to visiting travellers from a non-endemic area is much lower than in sub-Saharan Africa.

CHANGING ISSUES IN EPIDEMIOLOGY

The preceding sections have set out what can now be regarded as the classical theory of malaria epidemiology, as formulated by Macdonald (1950), building upon the foundations laid down by Ross. This is still a satisfying theory of the macro-epidemiology of malaria transmission and provides a broad explanation of the very different patterns of malaria seen in various endemic areas. It is repeated here as the necessary underpinning for clinicians, who may be unaware of this body of theory which helps to explain the clinical variation seen.

For those concerned with malaria control at specific sites, the more detailed computer-based model based on the Garki project in Nigeria (Molineaux and Gramiccia, 1980) is a refined version of the Macdonald model. It pays more attention to human acquired immunity and is of value in anticipating the likely effects of control measures, understanding seasonal transmission and guiding the timing and coverage of interventions aiming to limit transmission.

In recent years new observations have accumulated and new issues and approaches are emerging that are not readily understandable in terms of classical theory. Some observations fall outside classical theory because they stem from current interest in the epidemiology of malarial disease rather than transmission. Others are mainly concerned with the consequences of water resource development in Africa and the use of insecticide-impregnated bed nets in areas of stable transmission. A third set of data, on antigenic variation in relation to rates of antibody acquisition in human populations, has been used to support an alternative to the classical theory. These observations will be briefly described. The effects of genetic heterogeneity of people, vectors and parasites underlie several of these observations and hypotheses, and only now are the basic scientific tools becoming available to analyse this infraspecific variation. What currently appear as scattered anomalies should be incorporated into a more comprehensive theory in due course. Such a theory needs to encompass disease as well as infection and transmission, and proposals have already been put forward (Gupta et al, 1994c) although it is too early to assess their validity adequately.

It has long been known that malaria intensity is very patchily distributed. Thus, two villages in The Gambia (Keneba and Manduar) are quite near each other and yet have shown a markedly different parasite and spleen rate for over 40 years. In the early part of this period the area would have been considered holoendemic, with a great excess of transmission over that needed to infect everyone, so that one would have expected a comparable level of infection. Even in the forest zone of Sierra Leone, with very high transmission levels, there is intervillage variation in the intensity of human infection.

This variation is still more apparent under conditions of water resource development. The move from rainfed agriculture to irrigated rice growing in both West and East Africa results in an increase in mosquito populations, particularly in the dry season. Observations from The Gambia and from Burkina Faso have indeed documented the rise in anophelines but this has not been associated with increased malaria. The explanation may lie in different cytotypes within the An. gambiae complex having variable man-biting habits, or in a short mosquito adult life expectancy during the hot dry season preventing completion of the extrinsic cycle of malaria development, or in some other mechanism.

Of greater epidemiological interest are the results of trials of bed nets impregnated with pyrethroid insecticides. These have been shown to reduce markedly the incidence of clinical malaria in children and, to a lesser extent, the level of parasitaemia and parasite prevalence in first trials in The Gambia, where currently a child receives one or a few infective bites annually. This is most encouraging for control and is in line with theoretical expectations. However, subsequent trials in areas with a very high perennial transmission level, e.g. in Tanzania (with one infective bite nightly in Ifakara: Smith et al, 1993) and in Sierra Leone (with over 30 infective bites annually/person: Bockarie et al, 1994), have also shown a 50% reduction in clinical attacks of malaria (N. Marbiah, personal communication) and some decrease in parasitaemia that was less expected. It has been postulated that this is because of a reduced inoculum of sporozoites/infective bites, but there is no simple relation between inoculum size and clinical severity in malaria (Glynn and Bradley, 1995) and other statistical explanations may play a part (Glynn et al, 1994). The precise consequences of nets for parasitaemia need to be further defined, but if there is true dissociation between effects on parasitaemia and on clinical malaria, one explanation would point to genetic diversity in the pathogenicity of the falciparum malaria parasites.

With the renewed focus upon malarial disease rather than infection there have come efforts to standardize the definition of clinical malaria attacks. In areas of low transmission there is no problem as those who get infected usually become ill, as with travellers from the UK to malarious regions. But in holoendemic areas, where about 75% of children may be expected to have parasitaemia on any cross-sectional survey, the definition of a clinical malaria episode is fraught with difficulty. For practical purposes definition depends on a fever combined with a raised parasitaemia, but much effort has been devoted to determining the cut-off level of parasitaemia. This is certainly age- and place-dependent. Because small changes in the cut-off level have large effects on assessed clinical malaria incidence, other markers of clinical disease have been sought (Hurt et al, 1994). Circulating tumour necrosis factor (TNF) receptor levels remain raised for several hours after an attack, longer than TNF itself, but questions of specificity remain and other clinical markers are being actively sought. There seems no doubt that changes in transmission levels, induced by bed nets, can produce large changes in clinical malaria even under holoendemic conditions. One possible explanation would be genetic diversity in infecting parasites and variable strain-specific immunity in the hosts.

Recent observations in East Africa have shown marked differences in the pattern of severe malaria in childhood between two sites each with high transmission. Severe and sometimes life-threatening anaemia is a consequence of intense malaria infections in young children. Cerebral malaria tends to occur in slightly older children. Cerebral malaria is a major public health problem in one highly malarious area, yet in another anaemia is very prevalent in young children but cerebral malaria is rarely seen. The data of Erunkulu et al (1992) provides no support for the view that cerebral malaria only develops in those not previously exposed to infection.

Gupta et al (1994a,b) have attempted to explain these an
ings in a theoretical model that places great stress on antige
P. falciparum and implies that the parasite behaves as if th
different strains with little cross-immunity. Overall, malariai .
postulated to be a consequence of having acquired immunity to the may
of strains circulating locally. Severe childhood anaemia results from
sequential infections by many strains that have a cumulative destructive
effect on the red cells whilst cerebral malaria is proposed to be due to an
unusually pathogenic strain. In Papua New Guinea, Day et al (1992) and
Gupta et al (1994c) have shown that the prevalent immunity to particular
antigenic types builds up slowly over childhood and adolescence even
though immune responses to malaria parasites as a whole rise very fast
indeed (Day et al, 1992). This theory would also explain the effects of bed
nets upon clinical malaria attacks. A corollary of assuming that the antigenic strains behave separately in man is that estimates of the BCCR are
too high by a factor roughly equal to the number of parasite strains circulating. This lower BCRR is hard to square with the extreme difficulty of stopping malaria transmission in sub-Saharan Africa and also with the
observations in East Africa that suggest a large degree of mixing of antigenic strains during ookinete formation. The theory places great emphasis
on parasite genetic variation.

Other recent work by Kwiatkowski and colleagues, emphasizing the role
of TNF in the pathogenesis of severe malaria, has shown that Gambian
populations vary in their genetic capacity to produce high levels of TNF
and that this is a risk factor for severe malaria. The TNF2 allele occurs at a
gene frequency of 16% in a population where it is correlated with a seven-
fold increase in the risk of developing cerebral malaria, and must therefore
have compensating advantages (McGuire et al, 1994).

Recent epidemiological advances have therefore enabled malaria
epidemiology to begin to incorporate disease as well as transmission in its
purview. The previous concern with the population dynamics of vectors
and hosts has reached its limits and the genetic heterogeneity of malaria
parasites and of people is being opened up as the likely key to advances in
our understanding of this most important of human parasitic infections.

CHANGING EPIDEMIOLOGY

The picture of the pattern of malaria in the world, say before the Second
World War, that emerges is of risk throughout the tropics and much of the
sub-tropics including the Mediterranean littoral and southern USA, with a
few exceptions, notably the Polynesian and Micronesian islands of the
Pacific that lack anopheline mosquitoes, waterless deserts without
mosquito breeding places, and mountains whose elevation reduces the
temperature below that needed to maintain the extrinsic cycle of the malaria
parasite. This picture has subsequently been changed by four groups of
factors: (1) changes in the physical environment; (2) the consequences of

attempted malaria eradication; (3) the consequences of chemotherapy; and (4) current approaches to malaria control.

Changes in the environment

Environmental change has greatly affected malaria epidemiology, but not in simple or straightforward ways. Anopheline mosquitoes breed in fresh (a few species in brackish) water and each species has its own relatively rigid preferences for egg-laying and larval development. Most anophelines breed in clean (even if turbid) water and they do not flourish in water highly polluted by organic matter even though culicine mosquitoes may do well in polluted water. So anophelines tend to diminish under urban pollution, although *An. stephensi* flourishes in urban water impoundments and tanks in the Indian sub-continent and is a serious malaria vector.

The specificity of anopheline breeding habits can be deliberately exploited for malaria control. Habitats are altered to make them unfavourable to the previously ascertained local malaria vector, a process known as species sanitation and still applicable for local malaria control in endemic areas. But it is not universally applicable. *Anopheles gambiae*, in particular, breeds in temporary pools and puddles, even the rainwater collecting in an animal's hoofprint and because it can develop in a few days it is scarcely feasible to use environmental measures against it except in densely populated areas or plantation agriculture.

Environmental changes taking place for reasons unrelated to health may greatly affect malaria transmission. Water resource developments such as irrigation schemes may increase anopheline densities in areas of unstable malaria and lead to epidemics. So too may irrigation water in areas of seasonal transmission by creating a second peak of anophelines in the middle of the dry season, although in two areas of West Africa this was not accompanied by a second peak of malaria. Deforestation has complex effects. It brings people into contact with jungle mosquitoes. In the Amazon basin *An. darlingi* and in South East Asia *An. dirus* are both highly efficient malaria vectors and lead to intensified malaria among loggers and those working at the forest edge. But when the forest is completely destroyed the shaded breeding sites also go and the malaria risk falls again.

Environmental effects may interact with social and economic pressures in a complex way. Many malaria problems of South East Asia are related to a complex of issues in the forests that are predominantly located in hilly areas along international borders, often inhabited by ethnic minority groups who have some degree of alienation from the central governments. Consequently the malaria control services may operate inadequately, while the inhabitants may subsist by smuggling, illegal logging and gem mining, which bring them into the forest at night-time, when mosquitoes bite predominantly, under outdoor conditions without proper housing to protect them, and both logging and gem mining create new breeding places for the *An. dirus* and *An. minimus* mosquitoes of the forest and forest edge. Whilst in tropical Africa south of the Sahara malaria transmission may be general, in many parts of Asia and Latin America it is more a problem of those both economically and environmentally marginalized. In these areas the risk to the backpacking visitor 'off the beaten track' will be very much greater than to visitors who stay in resorts or capital cities.

There has been much concern that a consequence of global warming might be a substantial increase in the range and intensity of human malaria. The one aspect of transmission that is unequivocally temperature-dependent in a straightforward way is the duration of the extrinsic cycle (or incubation period in the mosquito) and it has been shown that a rise of, say, 2°C will have a large effect on the BCRR at the temperature limits of transmission (Bradley, 1993). However, the effects of increased temperature on mosquito survival and proliferation will depend on the humidity and rainfall changes, concerning which there is substantial uncertainty. Precise predictions are therefore difficult, though in general conditions for malaria transmission are likely to become more favourable as global warming occurs. However, this is unlikely to greatly affect the horizontal distribution of malaria as already the northern limit of malaria endemicity is kept far south of its natural level by deliberate action to control the disease. Only under anarchic conditions will malaria spread to its climate limits. The main effects of global warming will be seen in the highland areas of tropical countries such as Ethiopia, Kenya and Rwanda where the edge of malaria transmission will be pushed uphill into the densely populated mountains.

The consequences of attempted eradication

When DDT and other residual insecticides became available during the Second World War they transformed the approach to malaria control from a local environmental and personal protection activity into a community-wide reduction of transmission, because the anophelines resting in houses after feeding on people absorbed toxic doses of insecticide from sprayed walls which kept a deposit of insecticides for many months. This not only killed mosquitoes, but more particularly reduced their chances of reaching an advanced age (for a mosquito!) and dramatically reduced malaria transmission. The results were remarkable. In some Greek islands, transmission was effectively halted for 4 years. When spraying was stopped after this time, mosquitoes returned but malaria did not, as infections had meanwhile died out or been treated. This eradication of malaria, which first happened coincidentally, was then developed as a well-planned and time-limited onslaught on malaria, that if successful would permanently rid countries of the disease and the parasites (Pampana, 1963). It was pursued with great energy between 1950 and 1970 with the successful eradication of malaria from all of Europe, the USA, the USSR and many islands and other isolated foci. These remain risk-free, except for re-invasion of some of the former Soviet Central Asian Republics. At the other extreme, African countries south of the Sahara were little involved in attempts at eradication; resources and health services were inadequate and endemicity so high and stable that success would have been impossible. Greater efforts were made by countries at the southern edge of transmission (South Africa and parts of Zimbabwe) or where altitude made many parts either malaria-free or with unstable malaria, as in Ethiopia. Between the extremes, the vast malarious tracts of Asia, Latin America and Oceania were the object of huge efforts to eradicate malaria that were remarkably successful in almost stopping transmission, but which failed to get rid of the last cases over the succeeding decade. Since the drive to eradicate is inevitably time-limited, the programmes then collapsed and were followed by a resurgence of malaria in the face of demoralized control activities (Sharma and Mehrotra, 1986). The result is a substantial level of transmission in most of the less prosperous countries of South and South East Asia and of the Amazon basin, a much lower level in the Middle East and Central America, and very little residual malaria in North Africa and the Eastern Mediterranean littoral. However, many immigrants to Western Europe left South Asia at the height of efforts at eradication and many may not now realize that they, or their children, returning on holiday visits to friends and relations, are going to what are now highly malarious areas.

The consequences of chemotherapy

Until 1950, although there was some innate variation in the detailed susceptibility of malaria parasites to anti-malarial drugs, it could be assumed that the parasites were susceptible to the available drugs. This is no longer the case, and *P. falciparum*, in particular, has developed widespread resistance to the commoner anti-malarials. Resistance to pyrimethamine arose early, because it appears that the genes for resistance are present at a low level in natural populations of *P. falciparum*, and the selection pressure generated by the drug's use on a large scale for prophylaxis rapidly leads to resistance becoming widespread. The majority of *P. falciparum* populations in Africa and Asia are at least partly resistant to pyrimethamine.

Of much greater practical importance is resistance to chloroquine. This was first detected in the early 1950s in Colombia, and shortly afterwards on the Thai–Cambodia border. The subsequent data are compatible with spread of resistance from these two foci; mainly the Asian one, so that chloroquine resistance reached Africa 15 years ago and is now widespread through the areas of stable intense transmission. The intensity of chloroquine resistance varies from the level known as RI, where the parasites disappear from the blood after a standard treatment of chloroquine only to reappear after several days, through to RIII where the parasite density is little affected by a treatment dose of chloroquine. In broad terms, *P. falciparum* is highly resistant to chloroquine in South East Asia, resistance is present but less prominent in South Asia, and a high degree of resistance is also present in sub-Saharan Africa and the Amazon basin. Since chloroquine is the only inexpensive anti-malarial available on a large scale in developing countries, the epidemiology of severe morbidity and of mortality due to malaria is much affected by the level of chloroquine resistance in areas of high transmission, and the situation in Africa is rapidly deteriorating in this respect. However, even where chloroquine resistance is a major problem, many, usually the majority, of *P. falci-*

parum strains circulating in the community are still susceptible to chloro-quine.

Where other drugs have been used substantially for chemotherapy, resistance to these develops, and multiple drug resistance becomes prevalent, most notably in South East Asia, so that on the Cambodia–Thailand border up to 40% of clinical falciparum cases may be resistant to mefloquine, the most recently introduced, and expensive, anti-malarial.

The epidemiology of malaria throughout the world depends therefore on the environment as it affects the ecology of anopheline mosquitoes and the duration of the malaria parasites' extrinsic cycles. The anophelines have been affected over time by environmental changes (whether aimed at their control or for multiple other purposes or as side-effects of those purposes), and the anopheline populations and parasite populations by the attempts at malaria eradication and the use of chemotherapy in case management. The result is an extremely variable level of malaria endemicity, as measured by the BCRR, which differs a 1000-fold between different endemic areas and reaches its highest levels in tropical Africa. Regulation of transmission by acquired but incomplete immunity of the human hosts will limit the levels of transmission observed in endemic populations and the risk to non-immunes introduced into that population but this will still vary greatly, so that in the less highly endemic areas of Asia or at the edge of the Sahara a person may receive, on average, one infective mosquito bite/year, while in rural Tanzania the rate may reach an average of 1–10 infective bites/night.

Current approaches to malaria control

In the wake of attempts at eradication, malaria control has been of very variable standard in endemic countries, resulting in a patchy distribution of malaria incidence. Residual spraying with insecticides has been maintained in many Asian countries although coverage is usually low due to the protests of householders. So-called 'active case detection' by house visiting has also been maintained but is currently proving too demanding of resources. In spite of a renewed interest in biological and environmental control of vector breeding, efforts to implement this have so far been on a limited scale, though more substantial efforts are likely.

The main novel approach to control, in the absence of an operationally usable vaccine, has been the use of bed nets impregnated with pyrethroid insecticides. In principle this had the advantage over simple bed nets in that, even in the presence of a hole or somewhat defective use, mosquitoes would still not gain access or would die if they did, while the amount of insecticide needed was far less than for residual spraying of houses. Additionally, the impregnated net acts as a baited trap at night, as mosquitoes are attracted to the net by the carbon dioxide from the sleeping person and may then take up a lethal dose of insecticide. In controlled trials in highly endemic areas it was found that use of impregnated bed nets substantially reduced morbidity and clinical attacks due to malaria, while having a much smaller effect on the prevalence of parasitaemia. This pattern has been found in several African sites. Even in the forest zone of West

Africa with perennial transmission at a high level, the frequency of clinical malaria attacks in young children was reduced by 50% when impregnated bed nets were used. A national programme has been carried out in The Gambia and the method is being widely applied following successful trials in several countries of Asia, Africa and Oceania.

The main thrust of contemporary control has been set out by the World Health Organization and involves a shift from a primary emphasis on transmission control to the reduction of morbidity and mortality from malaria, with transmission control in selected circumstances, attempts to prevent or control epidemics of malaria, and a regular review of epidemiological data and plans for control. The key change has been towards reduction of disease rather than infection as such.

MALARIA EPIDEMIOLOGY IN TRAVELLERS FROM NON-ENDEMIC COUNTRIES

Whilst imported malaria into non-endemic countries comprises less than 0.01% of the world's malaria, the condition is sufficiently common in temperate countries that many doctors will encounter cases. Falciparum malaria is a medical emergency with a significant case mortality in non-immunes, so that its prevention, prompt detection and management are important in travellers. Appropriate measures depend upon understanding malaria epidemiology in travellers.

The pattern of imported malaria in temperate countries depends strongly on the scale of travel and the endemic countries visited. The risk to the individual traveller is a function of the place visited, the category of traveller and the precautions taken against infection. Both aspects will be illustrated with particular reference to UK data, which is more complete and more fully analysed than for many countries.

Imported malaria was at its lowest level in the mid 1960s for three main reasons: the massive increase in low cost air travel to the tropics had not yet occurred, no tropical wars involving European nationals on a large scale were taking place, and the world was closer to eradicating malaria than at any other time before or since, so the infectious reservoir was at its lowest. Since then, the amount of imported malaria has risen rapidly, often tending to stabilize by the 1990s. The detailed pattern varied by country. For example, in the UK, where less than 100 cases were imported (and reported) annually around 1970, there was a rapid rise to over 2000 cases/year before 1980 and the figure has remained around that level subsequently (Bradley, 1989). The initial rise was in vivax malaria, particularly from the Indian sub-continent. This was partly because *P. vivax*, having a shorter transmission cycle than *P. falciparum* at the same ambient temperature, led the resurgence of malaria in India and also because immigration from the sub-continent was at a high level and provided many cases of imported malaria. Vivax malaria reached a plateau in the 1980s. The immigrants had by now settled in the UK and an increasing proportion of the malaria cases from Asia was in settled immigrants or their descendants visiting friends and relations in the sub-continent. In recent years there has been a decrease in imported vivax malaria due to improved control within India.

By contrast, falciparum malaria has gradually and steadily increased in absolute numbers of cases as well as relative to vivax malaria, becoming the most commonly seen species from 1988. No section of the travelling community is free of risk, but most cases of falciparum malaria in the UK are among settled immigrants revisiting their countries of origin in Africa, in tourists and business travellers, and in foreign visitors falling ill while in the UK.

Because realizing possible risk is the key to early diagnosis and prompt treatment, the travel history of a patient with fever of an influenza-like illness is critical. Several aspects of risk are easily forgotten. No prophylactic measure will give 100% protection so there is always the possibility of malaria in those who have visited endemic areas. A businessman may say that he has visited New York but fail to mention that on a previous trip 2 weeks ago he was in Abidjan or Manaus. The person who has visited Australia may forget that his ticket allowed a 2 day stopover in a South East Asian country. Marginalized ethnic groups, especially illegal immigrants, have reasons to give inaccurate travel histories.

The determinants of malaria, whether in travellers to, or the indigenous inhabitants of, a country, are therefore diverse and the risk varies greatly. This will influence the choice of anti-malarial chemoprophylaxis for travellers, where the malaria risk has to be balanced against that of possible side-effects of the drug, but does not affect the need to minimize mosquito bites (Bradley, 1993). Moreover, since the risk to the non-immune of serious disease and death will be equally high once an infective bite for *P. falciparum* is received, the importance of a high index of suspicion, early diagnosis and prompt treatment cannot be over-emphasized.

SUMMARY

The initially very diverse epidemiology of malaria, with a thousandfold variation in transmission between different areas depending on anopheline mosquito biology, has been further complicated in the last two decades by the consequences of attempted eradication; by environmental change especially water resource developments, deforestation and re-afforestation, and urbanization; and by rapidly increasing resistance of falciparum malaria to successive antimalarial drugs but especially to chloroquine. Increased travel and forced migration has added to malaria in non-immune populations. Control strategies have been modified but, apart from the use of insecticide-impregnated bed nets, no new control methods have come into operational use recently.

REFERENCES

Bockarie MJ, Service MW, Barnish G et al (1994) Malaria in a rural area of Sierra Leone. III. Vector ecology and disease transmission. *Annals of Tropical Medicine and Parasitology* **88(3):** 251–262.

Brabin BJ (1983) An analysis of malaria in pregnancy in Africa. *Bulletin of the World Health Organization* **61**: 1005–1016.

Bradley DJ (1989) Current trends in malaria in Britain. *Journal of the Royal Society of Medicine* **82**: 8–13.

Bradley DJ (1993) Prophylaxis against malaria for travellers from the United Kingdom. *British Medical Journal* **306**: 1247–1252.

Davidson G (1955) Further studies of the basic factors concerned in the transmission of malaria. *Transactions of the Royal Society of Tropical Medicine and Hygiene* **49**: 339–350.

Day KP & Marsh K (1991) Naturally acquired immunity to *Plasmodium falciparum. Immunology Today* **12**: 68–71.

Day KP, Koella JC, Nee S et al (1992) Population genetics and dynamics of *Plasmodium falciparum*: an ecological view. *Parasitology* **(supplement) 104**: 35–52.

Erunkulu OA, Hill AV, Kwiatkowski DP et al (1992) *Severe Malaria in Gambian Children is Not Due to Lack of Previous Exposure to Malaria.* Banjul, The Gambia: MRC Laboratories.

Garnham PCC (1977) The continuing mystery of relapses in malaria. *Protozoological Abstracts* **1**: 1–12.

Garnham PCC (1988) Malaria parasites of man: life-cycles and morphology. In Wernsdorfer WH & MacGregor I (eds) *Malaria*, pp. 61–96. Edinburgh: Churchill Livingstone.

Garnham PCC, Bray RS, Bruce-Chwatt LJ et al (1975) A strain of *Plasmodium vivax* characterised by prolonged incubation; morphological and biological characteristics. *Bulletin of the World Health Organization* **52**: 21–32.

Glynn JR & Bradley DJ (1995) Inoculum size, incubation period and severity of malaria. Analysis of data from malaria therapy records. *Parasitology* **110**: 7–19.

Glynn JR, Lines JD & Bradley DJ (1994) Impregnated bednets and the dose-severity relationship in malaria. *Parasitology Today* **10**: 279–281.

Gupta S, Hill AV, Kwiatkowski et al (1994a) Parasite virulence and disease patterns in *Plasmodium falciparum* malaria. *Proceedings of the National Academy of Sciences of the United States of America* **91(9)**: 3715–3719.

Gupta S, Swinton J & Anderson RM (1994b) Theoretical studies of the effects of heterogeneity in the parasite population on the transmission dynamics of malaria. *Proceedings of the Royal Society of London Series B* **256**: 231–238.

Gupta S, Trenholme K, Anderson RM & Day KP (1994c) Antigenic diversity and the transmission dynamics of *Plasmodium falciparum. Science* **263**: 961–963.

Hurt N, Smith T, Tanner M et al (1994) Evaluation of C-reactive protein and haptoglobin as malaria episode markers in an area of high transmission in Africa. *Transactions of the Royal Society of Tropical Medicine and Hygiene* **88(2)**: 182–186.

Krotoski WA, Collins WE, Bray RS et al (1982) Demonstration of hypnozoites in sporozoite-transmitted *Plasmodium vivax* infection. *American Journal of Tropical Medicine and Hygiene* **31**: 1291–1293.

Macdonald G (1950) Community aspects of immunity to malaria. *British Medical Bulletin* **8**: 33–36.

Macdonald G (1952) The analysis of the sporozoite rate. *Tropical Diseases Bulletin* **49**: 569–585.

Macdonald G (1957) *The Epidemiology and Control of Malaria.* London: Oxford University Press.

McGuire W, Hill AV, Allsopp CE, Greenwood BM & Kwiatkowski D (1994) Variation in the TNF-alpha promoter region associated with susceptibility to cerebral malaria. *Nature* **371**: 508–510.

Miller LH, Mason SJ, Clyde DF & McGinniss MH (1976) The resistance factor to *Plasmodium vivax* in blacks. The Duffy blood group genotype, Fy Fy. *New England Journal of Medicine* **295**: 302–204.

Molineaux L & Gramiccia G (1980) *The Garki Project.* Geneva: World Health Organization.

Pampana EJ (1963) *A Textbook of Malaria Eradication.* London: Oxford University Press.

Phillips-Howard PA, Radalowicz A, Mitchell J, & Bradley DJ (1990) Risk of malaria in British residents returning from malarious areas. *British Medical Journal* **300**: 499–503.

Ross R (1910) *The Prevention of Malaria.* London: John Murray.

Sharma VP & Mehrotra KN (1986) Malaria resurgence in India: a critical study. *Social Science and Medicine* **22**: 835–845.

Smith T, Charlwood JD, Kihonda J et al (1993) Absence of seasonal variation in malaria parasitaemia in an area of intense seasonal transmission. *Acta Tropica* **54**: 55–72.

Targett GAT (ed.) (1991) *Malaria, Waiting for the Vaccine.* Chichester: Wiley.

2

Clinical immunology of malaria

MAY HO
MARY M. SEXTON

In the past decade, the intense research that has gone into the development of a malaria vaccine has provided new insight into many aspects of the interaction between *Plasmodium falciparum* and *P. vivax* and the human host. Among the most important is the recognition of the crucial role of cellular immune responses in both immunity to, and immunopathology caused by, these parasites. At the same time, the relevance of humoral responses has been re-emphasized. Furthermore, these advances have occurred against the background of the controversies surrounding the role of genetic regulation of the immune responses towards parasite antigens at the population level, and the importance of epitope polymorphism and antigenic variation as a means of immune evasion by the parasites. In this chapter, these recent developments in our understanding of the human immune responses to the two parasites will be reviewed. Immune responses to other human malaria parasites will be discussed where such information is available or relevant.

CLINICAL IMMUNOLOGICAL FEATURES

The complexity of the human immune response to infection by *P. falciparum* reflects the many antigens that the parasite presents to the host, in terms of stages in the life cycle and antigenic diversity, and their failure to establish immunological memory. As a result, natural immunity to infection develops slowly only upon repeated exposure, and is generally short-lived. In endemic areas, infants are protected from infection up to the age of 6 months, presumably due to the protective effect of maternal antibodies and the less favourable intracellular environment for parasite development (Bruce-Chwatt, 1952; Pasvol et al, 1976). Thereafter, the pattern of clinical disease and development of immunity are to a large extent determined by the level of malarial transmission. In hyperendemic areas, clinical malaria occurs mainly in children less than 1 year of age, and the major manifestation is anaemia (Brewster et al, 1990; Snow et al, 1994). There is a rapid decline in the rate of disease after the first year of life, as antimalarial immunity is acquired. Where transmission is less intense or seasonal, exposure is insufficient to induce significant immunity. As a result, individuals of all ages are susceptible to severe infection, but complications are especially evident in children from 1 to 4 years of age (Greenwood et al, 1987). Anaemia remains the main clinical manifestation in children of less than 1 year, while cerebral complications are seen in the older age groups. Whether the development of cerebral malaria among older children is related to lower previous exposure remains to be determined. In one study in The Gambia, children who developed cerebral malaria were found to have comparable prior exposure compared to control children, as judged by antibody responses to multiple parasite antigens and the ability of the antibodies to agglutinate a number of parasite isolates (Erunkulu et al, 1992). Protection against cerebral malaria in this population is believed to be linked to human leukocyte antigen (HLA)-B53 and against malarial anaemia to an HLA class II haplotype (DRB1*1302–DQB1*0501: Hill et al, 1991). Adults in hyperendemic areas are mostly asymptomatic, although there is some loss of immunity with increased prevalence of infection and severity of disease during pregnancy, particularly in primigravidae (McGregor, 1984). However, congenital malaria is rare.

IMMUNE RESPONSES TO SPOROZOITES

As early as the 1970s, irradiated sporozoites of P. falciparum and P. vivax were known to induce protective immunity in a high proportion of immunized volunteers (Clyde et al, 1973, 1975). Based on these results, and the observation, in vitro, that sporozoites were immobilized and rendered non-infective by antibodies against the circumsporozoite (CS) protein (Hollingdale et al, 1984), the first generation of P. falciparum vaccines was developed using an immunodominant B cell epitope $(NANP)_n$ from the conserved central repeat region of the CS protein. The failure of these vaccines to protect more than 20% of the vaccinees in several clinical trials (Ballou et al, 1987; Herrington et al, 1987; Fries et al, 1992) underscored for the first time the importance of the participation of T cells in protective immunity, both in providing memory and enhancement of antibody production, as well as in cell-mediated cytotoxicity. Subsequently, CD8+ cytotoxic T cells against the P. falciparum CS protein and its peptides have been demonstrated in previously infected individuals, although the presence and frequency of these cells differ in different study populations (Doolan et al, 1991, 1993; Sedegah et al, 1992). In mice, these cytotoxic cells recognize parasite antigenic determinants that are expressed on the surface of infected hepatocytes (Weiss et al, 1990). Cytotoxicity is at least partially mediated through interferon-γ (IFN-γ) (Ferreira et al, 1986), but interleukin 6 (IL-6) also appears to play a role (Pied et al, 1991).

Both the helper and cytotoxic T cell antigenic sites of the CS protein of P. falciparum occur outside the conserved central repeat region, and exhibit considerable epitope polymorphism (Good et al, 1988). However, within a certain geographical location, sequence variation is often limited (Yoshida et al, 1990; Doolan et al, 1992). Thus, the geographically restricted hetero-geneity of T cell epitopes appears unlikely to contribute to the slow development of immunity to sporozoites. This observation suggests that it may be feasible to develop a polyvalent vaccine consisting of a small number of CS peptides. Epitope polymorphism of the CS protein, includ-ing the central repeat region, has also been described for *P. vivax*, but its importance awaits studies on parasite population dynamics in different endemic locations (Qari et al, 1992).

Immune responses to the CS protein of *P. falciparum* and *P. vivax*, and overlapping peptides spanning the entire protein, have been studied extensively in different populations (Hoffman et al, 1989; Riley et al, 1990; Wongsrichanalai et al, 1991; Doolan et al, 1994). The detection of anti-bodies and/or cellular responses in the absence of clinical malaria in these studies is often equated with protection. The results should be interpreted with greater caution, as responsiveness or unresponsiveness in many of the studies were based largely on data obtained at a single point in time, and immune responses are known to vary with a number of factors, including the intensity of malarial transmission and concurrent infections at the time of study (Riley and Greenwood, 1990). There is, however, one consistent finding in these studies. Both cellular and antibody responses to the CS protein are present in only a proportion of exposed individuals, and are not invariably boosted by natural infection. Furthermore, responses to *P. falci-parum* CS protein are transient, being lost between 6 months (Webster et al, 1989) and 2 years after infection (Zevering et al, 1994). The duration of immunological memory appears to be much more prolonged after *P. vivax* infection, which suggests that antigenic persistence, presumably as hypno-zoites in the liver, may be necessary for its maintenance. However, since individuals are susceptible to multiple *P. vivax* infections, the relationship between T cell memory to CS peptides and protection needs to be clarified.

Other studies have demonstrated that CD4+ T cells of non-exposed indi-viduals also respond to some of the CS peptides (Zevering et al, 1992), and the phenotype of the responding cells (CD45RO+) suggests they have been previously activated by cross-reacting organisms. The cross-reactivity is much more evident against *P. falciparum* than *P. vivax* antigens. These T cells can be present in high frequencies and are clearly non-protective. In this way, cross-reactive organisms have the potential to bias the repertoire of sporozoite-responsive T cells and adversely affect the induction of protective immunity. This situation has been compared to the concept of 'original antigenic sin' or the immunological imprinting described for the influenza virus which has the ability to divert the antibody response to a second challenging strain towards cross-reactive epitopes (Good et al, 1993). Whether this results from a flaw in the immune system, or is a parasite-induced effect, remains to be determined. A variation of the same phenom-enon has recently been reported by Riley (1994) with regard to the antibody and lymphoproliferative responses to the blood stage merozoite surface antigen 1 (MSP-1). In this case, it was found that the patterns of antibody production or T cell reactivities in individuals living in an endemic area over long periods of time do not reflect exposure to multiple variants and strains.

Immune responses are always directed towards the same peptides, as if there is clonal dominance of initially recruited B and T cells so that the responses upon restimulation are only poorly cross-reactive with new variants.

The finding in mice that genes mapping to the major histocompatibility complex (MHC) are crucial for immune responses to the CS protein and defined peptide epitopes of *P. falciparum* raised great concern that genetically regulated non-responsiveness may be widespread in human populations (Good et al, 1990). This fear was reinforced by limited epidemiological studies (de Groot et al, 1989; Quakyi et al, 1989), which attributed unresponsiveness at a single time point to a genetic mechanism. Studies with a more careful follow-up have since shown that there is little evidence in humans of an association between HLA class II genotype and both humoral and cellular immune responses to the CS and other malaria proteins (Riley et al, 1992). However, some differences in response were observed among different ethnic groups, which suggests that genetic regulation which is not MHC-dependent may have a role.

From the foregoing account, it is clear that the mechanisms of protection against sporozoites are far more complex in humans than suggested by in vitro results and experimental models. Current research efforts in vaccine development include the identification and incorporation of T cell epitopes, optimization of the method of delivery of the CS peptides and boosting of their ability to induce cytotoxic T cells. The important question remains whether protection against malaria can be achieved through anti-sporozoite immunity.

IMMUNE RESPONSES TO ASEXUAL PARASITES

Although asexual *P. falciparum* parasites are not the initial stage of the parasite to be encountered by the host, naturally acquired immunity to malaria appears to be directed towards this stage of the life cycle. This immunity is manifested in individuals who harbour a low-grade parasitaemia with no clinical symptoms. Asexual blood-stage parasites are also responsible for most, if not all, of the disease manifestations. This observation led Sinton et al (1931) to hypothesize that immunity to *P. falciparum* infection is partly anti-parasitic and partly antitoxic, a position which has recently been re-stated as the dichotomy between anti-parasite and anti-disease immunity (Playfair et al, 1990). The revival of interest in such a concept is due to the demonstration of elevated levels of tumour necrosis factor (TNF-α), IL-1 and IL-6 in severe falciparum malaria (Grau et al, 1989; Kwiatkowski et al, 1990). Parasite exoantigens which are secreted into the culture supernatant stimulate production of TNF-α, and are shown to contain phospholipid (Bate et al, 1992). Immunization with these phospholipid-containing antigens have resulted in inhibition of TNF-α production in a murine model (Bate et al, 1993). Such inhibitory activity is also seen in acutely infected patients, and appears to be mediated by phosphatidylinositol-specific IgM. (Bate and Kwiatkowski, 1994). Antigens in a crude schizont lysate (Picot et al, 1990) and recombinant ring-infected erythrocyte surface antigen (Pf155/RESA: Picot et al, 1993) are also effective in inducing TNF-α production, which suggests that there may be more antigens than glycolipids involved in producing the disease manifestations of falciparum malaria.

While humoral responses may be sufficient for anti-disease immunity, both humoral and cell-mediated mechanisms have been implicated in anti-parasitic immunity against asexual *P. falciparum* parasites. Effective control of parasitaemia in all likelihood represents these two arms of the immune response working in concert. Perhaps the most convincing evidence for the role of antibodies in protection against malaria is that in endemic areas infants up to 6 months old are generally protected against infection, suggesting a vital role for maternal antibodies (Bruce-Chwatt, 1952). However, antibodies from the infant or cellular mechanisms may be operative even at this stage of life, as in utero sensitization to malarial antigens has been demonstrated (Desowitz et al, 1993). Additional evidence for the importance of antibodies in protection against infection with malaria comes from studies in which γ-globulin or purified placental IgG from immune adults was transfused into non-immune children during acute attacks of malaria, resulting in marked declines in parasitaemia (Cohen et al, 1961; Sabchareon et al, 1991). In the earlier study, antibodies were thought to agglutinate merozoites and thus inhibit reinvasion. More recent data obtained with purified IgG indicate that antibodies promote phago-cytosis of merozoites and, to a lesser degree, schizont-infected erythrocytes by monocytes (Bouharoun-Tayoun et al, 1990). The isotype and subclass of antibodies therefore becomes of critical importance, since IgG_2 and IgM are unable to arm monocytes, and may in fact inhibit opsonization by cytophilic antibodies. The observation that some individuals with high levels of anti-malarial antibodies may develop clinical symptoms can now be explained by the functional differences which exist among antibodies of the same antigenic specificity (Bouharoun-Tayoun and Druilhe, 1992). The relevance of these observations to immunity against blood-stage *P. falciparum* parasites has been demonstrated in an endemic population in which an imbalance of immunoglobulin production was noted. It was shown that IgM and IgG_2 predominated in susceptible groups while the increase in IgG_1 and IgG_3 with age correlated with clinical immunity.

Opsonized merozoites or parasitized erythrocytes can be phagocytosed by mononuclear phagocytes and trigger the intracellular generation of reactive oxidative intermediates. Alternatively, non-opsonized trophozoite- or schizont-infected erythrocytes can initiate the extracellular production of reactive oxygen intermediates by adherence via the CD36 molecule (Ockenhouse et al, 1989). This process is augmented by IFN-γ but down-regulated by IL-4 (Kumaratilake and Ferrante, 1992). There is also evidence that nitric oxide derivatives can mediate parasite destruction in a cell-free system (Rockett et al, 1991). However, it is difficult to implicate a role for nitric oxide in vivo as it is not produced by human mononuclear phagocytes (Murray and Teitelbaum, 1992), although endothelial cells may do so. Paradoxically, there is impairment of macrophage function after ingestion of *P. falciparum*-infected erythrocytes or isolated malarial pigment (Schwarzer et al, 1992). Iron released from malarial pigment in the monocyte phagolysosome may be responsible for the impairment of further phagocytic activity and oxidative burst.

Two other effector cells in addition to monocytes have been described. Neutrophils have been shown to phagocytose intraerythrocytic parasites of all stages and free merozoites, a process which is greatly enhanced by opsonization with antibody and complement (Kumaratilake et al, 1992). Killing by the respiratory burst is in turn augmented by TNF-α, IFN-γ and, less effectively, by lymphotoxin (Kumaratilake et al, 1991). Unlike the anti-plasmodial effect of macrophages, this killing activity is not downregulated by IL-4 (Kumaratilake and Ferrante, 1992). The participation of T cell cytokines in neutrophil-mediated parasite killing suggests that the anti-malarial activity of neutrophils is under T cell regulation.

Natural killer (NK) cells also appear to have cytolytic effect against schizonts, and the action is enhanced by the addition of IFN-γ or IL-2 (Orago and Facer, 1991). In acutely infected patients, there is a decrease in the CD56+ and CD16+ subsets of NK cells, which is accompanied by an impairment of the ability to lyse intraerythrocytic parasites. Interestingly, asymptomatic individuals have the highest levels of CD56+ NK cells with an enhanced response to cytokines. NK cells may constitute a first-line defense against P. falciparum parasites before T cells are activated. NK cells may also be a major source of IFN-γ, which would in turn enhance macrophage function.

A seminal report by Grun and Weidanz (1981) showed that B cell-deficient chickens were able to clear a P. gallinaceum parasitaemia. The observation was recently confirmed in a definitive mouse model against P. chabaudi chabaudi and P. vinckeii petteri infection (van der Heyde et al, 1994). These findings imply the involvement of antibody-independent T cell mechanisms for parasite removal in these experimental models. The relevance of T cell-mediated immunity towards blood-stage P. falciparum parasites remains to be determined. Two recent developments suggest anti-parasitic roles for both γδ T cells and αβ T cells.

γδ T cells constitute a minor subset (< 5%) of T cells that express the γ and δ chains of the T cell receptor. They have been shown to display non-MHC-restricted cytotoxicity towards certain tumour cell lines (Porcelli et al, 1991) and are responsive to mycobacterial antigens and heat shock proteins (Kabelitz et al, 1990). These cells are markedly elevated in the peripheral blood and spleen of patients with acute P. falciparum malaria as a result of polyclonal activation (Ho et al, 1994). The increase in γδ T cells is characteristically noted following the start of treatment, and may persist for up to 3–4 months. The antigen specificity of these γδ T cells is difficult to demonstrate in short term cultures (Ho et al, 1994), but they respond to schizont antigens when cultured for several weeks (Roussilhon et al, 1994). Furthermore, γδ T cell clones obtained from immune donors appear to be cytotoxic to autologous αβ T cell clones specific for the same malarial extract, suggesting a role for γδ T cells in the regulation of αβ T lymphocyte-mediated response to the parasite (Roussilhon et al, 1994).

Recently, human γδ T cell clones have been shown to inhibit replication of blood-stage *P. falciparum* in vitro in a dose-dependent manner (Elloso et al, 1994). Morphologically there does not appear to be any inhibition of development from rings to schizonts. The targets recognized are believed to be merozoites, and contact between the merozoites and γδ T cells is required for inhibition of parasite growth. The γδ T cell clones used in these studies are not malaria antigen-specific, and do not require any accessory cells. Furthermore, there is no increase in killing after stimulation with malarial antigens. In contrast, malaria-specific CD4+ and CD8+ T cells, which also appear to inhibit parasite growth, require the presence of adherent cells, and the inhibition is augmented by stimulation with specific antigen (Fell et al, 1994).

Elevation of γδ T cells has also been observed during clinical paroxysms of *P. vivax* malaria, as well as between paroxysm and during convalescence of patients with severe infection (Perera et al, 1994). The increase in γδ T cells was associated with gastrointestinal symptoms such as nausea, anorexia and vomiting. No increase was seen in patients with mild infection. The conclusion that γδ T cells contribute to the pathology of *P. vivax* infection, in particular gastrointestinal pathology, appears somewhat premature without stricter definition of disease severity in *P. vivax* malaria.

In both humoral and cell-mediated immunity, immune responses against blood-stage *P. falciparum* parasites are largely directed towards antigens expressed on the surface of infected erythrocytes, and may be complicated by antigenic variation. In *P. falciparum*-infected erythrocytes, antigenic variation has been demonstrated using microagglutination. Sera from convalescent Gambian children agglutinate only the homologous parasite isolate, whereas sera from immune adults agglutinate a number of parasite isolates, suggesting previous exposure to a number of variant strains (Marsh and Howard, 1986). Antigenic variation has also been demonstrated in *P. vivax*-infected erythrocytes (Mendis et al, 1988). However, the microagglutination assay does not distinguish between antigenic variation, i.e. the variation of the antigenic phenotype of a specific surface molecule at the clonal level, and antigenic diversity created by multiple different stable alleles within a mixed population of organisms. To further address this issue, studies were performed with cloned parasites which showed that the clones display differences in their agglutination by clone-specific antisera (Biggs et al, 1991; Roberts et al, 1992). Moreover, the clonal variation appears to involve P. falciparum erythrocyte membrane protein (PfEMP1), the putative parasite ligand which mediates cytoadherence, and results in modulation of the endothelial receptor phenotypes. The variation occurs in the absence of immune pressure at a rate of 2.4% per life cycle, which suggests it may be genetically determined as in the case of *P. fragile* in its natural host, *Macaca sinica* (Handunnetti et al, 1987).

IMMUNOPATHOLOGY

Three major immunological abnormalities have been observed in patients with acute falciparum malaria. The first is a failure of lymphoproliferation in vitro in response to malaria-specific antigens (Ho et al, 1986). In patients with severe disease, the immune unresponsiveness extends to unrelated antigens such as purified protein derivatives and streptococcal antigens. At the same time, there are markedly elevated levels of the inflammatory cytokines TNF α, IL-1 and IL-6 which have been positively correlated with morbidity and mortality (Grau et al, 1989; Kwiatkowski et al, 1990). This subject will be discussed in Chapter 9: The biology of malarial fever. There is also evidence of intense T cell activation, as indicated by elevated levels of soluble IL-2 receptor, CD4 and CD8 (Ho et al, 1988, 1990; Jakobsen et al, 1994).

The mechanisms of antigen-specific immune unresponsiveness have been investigated extensively in several laboratories. Results differ with regard to alterations in the CD4/CD8 T cell ratio, and the role of CD8+ and adherent suppressor cells (Troye-Blomberg et al, 1984; Ho et al, 1986, 1988; Riley et al, 1989). The discrepancies may reflect differences in the patient populations with respect to the level of transmission and the extent of previous exposure to P. falciparum. The one consistent finding was of a defect in IL-2 production and IL-2 receptor expression which, at least in our hands, was not convincingly reversed by the addition of exogenous human IL-2 (Ho et al, 1988).

Several clinical observations appear to be a direct result of the immuno-suppression seen in P. falciparum malaria. A poor response to the O antigen of Salmonella typhi and to tetanus toxoid has been reported in acutely infected children (Greenwood et al, 1972). Further studies in young Nigerian children showed that, among the common childhood immuniza-tions, the suppressive effect of malaria is limited to meningococcal poly-saccharide vaccine which is known to be poorly immunogenic in that age group (Bradley-Moore et al, 1985). Perhaps a more pertinent question to ask is whether a patent parasitaemia will suppress response to a malaria vaccine, an issue which needs to be addressed in current vaccine trials in the field.

Immunosuppression is also thought to predispose infected individuals to concomitant infections. However, this does not appear to pose a major clinical problem. In adult Thai patients, concomitant bacterial infection is seen in less than 10% of patients with cerebral malaria (NJ White et al, unpublished data). In The Gambia, children with salmonella septicaemia are more likely to have a recent history of malaria (Marsh and Greenwood, 1986), while Oppenheimer et al (1986) observed an association between malaria and other infections, particularly those of the lower respiratory tract, among children in Papua New Guinea.

The correlation of intense T cell activation with disease severity suggests that T cell cytokines may play an important role in the pathogenesis of severe falciparum malaria. Recent studies show that of the four T cell cytokines IL-2, IL-4, IL-10 and IFN-γ, IFN-γ and IL-10 are consistently produced in vivo by patients suffering from uncomplicated and severe falciparum malaria, and are significantly higher in patients with severe disease (Peyron et al, 1994; Ho et al, in press). IL-2 is not produced, similar to the situation in vitro, and IL-4 production is within normal limits.

Furthermore, IFN-γ augments, while IL-10 completely inhibits, TNF-α production by peripheral blood mononuclear cells in response to malaria antigen in vitro. These results indicate that in addition to the inflammatory cytokines, the course of *P. falciparum* infection is influenced by cytokines that may have no direct pathological effects but are nevertheless important regulators of the immune responses to the parasite.

In addition to the modulation of cellular responses, *P. falciparum* malaria is also associated with autoantibody production and complement activation. Autoantibodies to a number of self antigens have been described in acutely infected patients, including anti-nuclear, anti-DNA, anti-red cell, anti-smooth muscle and anti-cardiolipin antibodies. However, these antibodies are rarely of pathogenic consequence except in the case of antibodies against triosephosphate isomerase, which have been implicated in the persistent haemolysis following parasite clearance in a certain proportion of patients (Ritter et al, 1993). Of possibly greater importance is the interpretation of a positive result for autoantibodies in the context of malaria. In a recent study of 351 West Africans with malaria, tuberculosis or hepatitis B and normal controls, 7% of the normal controls were positive for anti-nuclear antibodies with several staining patterns, and 30.3% for anti-cardiolipin antibodies (Adebajo et al, 1993). Among patients with malaria, there was twice that frequency of anti-nuclear antibodies. Anti-neutrophil cytoplasmic antibodies were found in a few cases. The occurrence of at least anti-nuclear and anti-smooth muscle antibodies is not determined or influenced by racial differences (Daniel-Ribeiro et al, 1991). The findings suggest that extreme caution is required in the interpretation of autoantibody results in individuals from, or living in, the tropics, as well as in patients with tropical infections.

Complement is activated predominantly through the classical pathway in falciparum malaria (Phanuphak et al, 1985). Hypocomplementaemia is associated with the occurrence of cryoglobulins and circulating immune complexes. However, there is no convincing evidence that complement activation or immune complexes have a pathological role in acute malaria. In contrast to findings in a murine model, immune complexes do not inhibit Fc-receptor-mediated clearance of IgG-coated erythrocytes in patients with acute falciparum malaria (Ho et al, 1991).

ROLE OF THE SPLEEN

Regardless of the effector mechanism against intraerythrocytic *P. falciparum* parasites, the site of parasite destruction remains controversial. Although the spleen has been shown to be absolutely essential for host defense in animal models (Wyler et al, 1983), a recent report from Thailand suggests that splenectomized patients do not necessarily have a defect in parasite clearance or develop more severe disease (Looareesuwan et al, 1993). Radiolabelled clearance studies in these patients indicate that heat-damaged erythrocytes, which have rheological properties similar to parasitized erythrocytes, are sequestered in the liver and are removed at the same rate as in eusplenic individuals. In autopsy studies of the human spleen, phagocytosis of predominantly ring-infected erythrocytes is observed (Pongpanratn et al, 1989), and splenic sinusoids are not packed with crisis forms as would be expected if there had been significant extracellular oxidative killing.

The clearance of heat-damaged and antibody-coated erythrocytes has been studied in patients with acute falciparum malaria (Looareesuwan et al, 1987a; Ho et al, 1991). In the case of antibody-coated erythrocytes, there is a highly significant direct correlation between the clearance half-time and haematocrit on admission. The inverse correlation between clearance half-time and parasitaemia is equally significant. Collectively, these findings suggest that splenic clearance of sensitized erythrocytes contributes to the development of anaemia, while splenic clearance function may be impaired in patients who have higher parasitaemias. With both cell types, there is augmentation of the clearance process after the start of anti-malarial treatment. This may be analogous to the rapid clearance at crisis seen in *Plasmodium berghei* infected rats, and suggests an 'opening up' of the blood–spleen barrier as hypothesized by Weiss et al (1986). The clearance of heat-damaged erythrocytes is facilitated by splenomegaly while the size of the spleen has no effect on the clearance of IgG-sensitized cells. Splenic clearance function remains accelerated during convalescence, and is still evident in some patients four weeks after the start of treatment. The hyperactivity of the spleen almost certainly contributes to the shortened red cell survival that has been demonstrated in convalescent patients (Looareesuwan et al, 1987b).

IMMUNE RESPONSE TO SEXUAL PARASITES

Parasitaemic individuals, whether ill or asymptomatic, represent a reservoir of infectivity in a community due to their production of gametocytes. The conditions which promote development of gametocytes from merozoites remain unclear. In holoendemic areas, children under the age of 10 constitute approximately 70% of the infective pool (Boudin et al, 1991; Githeko et al, 1992). Immunity to sexual stages of the parasite, though of no immediate benefit to the host, can prevent transmission of disease by blocking the parasite life cycle within the mosquito.

Two general types of effector mechanisms against gametocytes have been described. Antibodies which inhibit the further development of extracellular sexual stages within the mosquito midgut are produced in response to infection with *P. falciparum* and *P. vivax*. In Papua New Guinea, where a high transmission rate of *P. falciparum* and *P. vivax* occurs, the frequency of transmission-blocking antibodies to *P. falciparum* is low (Graves et al, 1988). In contrast, 90% of people experiencing their second or third bout of infection with *P. vivax* in Sri Lanka produce antibodies which reduce the infectivity of mosquitoes (Mendis et al, 1987). The effect is most pronounced in the presence of complement. Paradoxically, certain infected individuals developed antibodies which enhanced the infectivity of *P. vivax* gametocytes (Gamage-Mendis et al, 1992). An enhancing effect is seen at low antibody titres, while a blocking effect occurred when antibodies reached higher levels. In contrast to immunity to sporozoites and asexual blood-stage parasites, transmission-blocking immunity is inversely correlated with age. Furthermore, immunological memory for transmission-blocking immunity appears to be transient (< 4 months) if present at all.

An effector mechanism that mediates the death of blood-stage *P. vivax* gametocytes but does not involve antibodies has also been described (Karunaweera et al, 1993). It involves TNF-α working in conjunction with as yet unidentified but essential serum factors. More recently, Naotunne et al (1993) demonstrated that the inhibitory effect of these mediators on *P. falciparum* and *P. vivax* gametocytes in vitro could be partially reversed by the nitric oxide synthase inhibitor N^GL-monomethyl arginine acetate, thus implicating the participation of leukocytes which release nitric oxide in the process. As pointed out earlier, this hypothesis is difficult to reconcile with the current view that neither human neutrophils nor monocytes produce nitric oxide under experimental conditions. The inhibitory activity is absent in semi-immune individuals, presumably due to the presence of antibodies that neutralize antigens which would have stimulated the production of parasite-killing factors.

SPECIAL CONSIDERATIONS

There are several clinical situations in which an aberrant immune response to malaria has resulted in established disease syndromes, while in others the effect of malaria on the underlying immunological status of the host is still a matter of speculation. These will be reviewed below.

Quartan malarial nephropathy

The frequency of the nephrotic syndrome in many parts of Africa is about 100 times greater than in Europe and America, and the condition appears to be a peculiar feature of *P. malariae* infection, which otherwise runs a relatively benign chronic course. In a clinicopathological study of 100 consecutive patients with childhood nephrotic syndrome in northern Nigeria, 20% was found to be due to quartan malarial nephropathy (Abdurrahman et al, 1990). Nephropathy is initiated by the deposition of *P. malariae* antigen–antibody complexes in the renal glomerular basement membrane (Hendrickse et al, 1977). Immunohistochemical staining shows granular deposits of mainly IgM and C3, and *P. malariae* antigen can be detected in about one-third of all biopsies. Tragically for the affected children, treatment of the infection and prevention of reinfection with anti-malarial chemoprophylaxis does not change the course of the condition which progresses relentlessly to chronic renal failure. Only a few patients respond to steroids or to azathioprine. The resistance to specific treatment suggests that the mechanism of renal damage may in fact be autoimmunity that has been triggered by cross-reacting parasite antigens. As the disease progresses, the histology changes from a granular to a diffuse glomerular staining pattern, similar to that produced by anti-basement membrane antibody. Why nephropathy develops only in *P. malariae* infection, and why the vast majority of those infected have no renal pathology, is not known.

Hyperreactive malarial splenomegaly

Hyperreactive malarial splenomegaly (HMS), previously known as the tropical splenomegaly syndrome, represents another aberrant immunological response to malarial parasites. In this condition, there is marked elevation of serum IgM levels and massive splenomegaly with resultant hypersplenism and pancytopenia. There is increased susceptibility to infection and increased mortality. Although malarial parasites are rarely demonstrable in the blood, the spleen size regresses and symptoms resolve with effective anti-malarial prophylaxis.

It is not known whether HMS results from an unusual pattern of malarial infection or from immune incompetence of the host. Family studies in Papua New Guinea, where HMS is common, suggest that a major sex-linked gene controls hyperreactivity to malaria (Serjeantson and Crane, 1991). At the cellular level, the hypergammaglobulinaemia is believed to be the result of uncontrolled polyclonal B cell activation in the absence of adequate numbers of CD8+ suppressor T cells (Hoffman et al, 1984) which have been depleted by an antibody-dependent cytotoxic mechanism (Piessens et al, 1985). In a subgroup of HMS patients who became resistant to anti-malarial treatment, clonal rearrangements of the Jh region of the immunoglobulin gene have been demonstrated (Bates et al, 1991). This finding suggests that clonal lymphoproliferation in these patients may evolve into a malignant proliferative disorder such as chronic lymphocytic leukaemia.

Burkitt's lymphoma

Burkitt's lymphoma, first described among Ugandan children in 1958, is a highly malignant B cell tumour which occurs in children living in hyperendemic malarial regions (endemic Burkitt's lymphoma), as well as in patients with AIDS and other immunodeficiency states. The aetiology of endemic Burkitt's lymphoma includes three inter-related factors. First, the ubiquitous Epstein–Barr virus (EBV) possesses oncogenic potential when it infects infants or very young children. Second, *P. falciparum* infection specifically depresses cytotoxic T cells controlling the polyclonal proliferation of EBV-infected B cells in the host (Whittle et al, 1984) which occurs as a result of infection of normal B cells by viruses liberated from infected cells (Lam et al, 1991). In addition, cell lines derived from EBV-carrying Burkitt's lymphoma often show an overall decrease in MHC class I antigen expression, and selective down-regulation of certain HLA-A and HLA-C alleles (Masucci and Klein, 1991). As a consequence, these malignant cells are often resistant to cytotoxic T lymphocyte-mediated destruction. Third, malignant changes occur when chromosomal translocations activate the cmyc oncogene which in turn induces uncontrolled B cell proliferation. Recent investigations indicate that Burkitt's lymphoma consists of several subtypes, defined by their clinical and molecular features (Magrath et al, 1992). The subtypes are environmentally determined, the rate of EBV association being highest in tropical Africa. It has been proposed that the pattern of infection (e.g. malaria) to which the young child is exposed influences the tumour subtype distribution by altering the relative and absolute numbers of various B cell precursors at sites of B cell ontogeny (the bone marrow and possibly mesentery). These B cells precursors are then susceptible to the specific chromosomal translocations associated with Burkitt's lymphoma.

Human immunodeficiency virus (HIV) infection and malaria

The commonest presentation of acquired immune deficiency syndrome (AIDS) in Africa is enteropathic AIDS with chronic watery diarrhoea and profound weight loss (Fleming, 1990). Infections which are known to require cell-mediated immunity such as *Mycobacterium tuberculosis* and *Toxoplasma gondii* occur at later stages of HIV infection when the number of CD4+ T cells drops below critical levels. This appears not to be the case with *P. falciparum* malaria. Many studies have shown that the prevalence or degree of parasitaemia of falciparum malaria is not significantly affected by concurrent HIV infection in infants (Greenberg et al, 1991), adult males (Muller and Moser, 1990) or women of childbearing age (Allen et al, 1991). Moreover, malaria infection does not appear to accelerate the progression of HIV-1 infection to AIDS.

The lack of any adverse effect of malaria on the progression of HIV infection is not surprising, since malaria is an acute febrile illness in which immunological abnormalities are readily reversible during convalescence. In hyperendemic areas, children suffer from at most three to four malaria attacks per year, but are more likely to have a single episode (Greenwood et al, 1987). The lack of effect of HIV infection on the incidence and severity of malaria on the other hand, raises questions regarding the import-ance of CD4+ T cells in protection against *P. falciparum* parasites. Various hypotheses have been proposed to explain the apparent inconsistency (Butcher, 1992). There appears to be selective depletion of T cell subsets expressing specific T cell receptor Vβ variants in HIV infection (Imberti et al, 1991). These cells may not be important in the immune response against malarial antigens. Also, killing of malarial parasites may be preserved in HIV infection as macrophages can be stimulated by parasite antigens to produce TNF-α in a T-independent fashion (Bate et al, 1992). Furthermore, the anti-parasitic effect of T cells in vivo may be due primarily to γδ T cells, the majority of which is CD4– CD8–. The intriguing possibility is that if the severity of malaria infection is related to an exaggerated T cell response, as suggested by in vitro data (see Immunopathology, above), then perhaps a reduction in CD4+ T cells would be beneficial to the host. This hypothesis is consistent with the lack of increased severity of cerebral malaria in HIV-positive patients (Niyongabo et al, 1994).

Malaria and pregnancy

Malaria is up to 12 times more common in pregnant women compared with their non-pregnant counterparts (McGregor, 1984). The infection is associated with increases in spontaneous abortion, stillbirths and low birth weight (Brabin, 1983). In areas of intense transmission, these adverse effects of falciparum malaria are largely confined to first pregnancies (McGregor, 1984). In areas of lower or unstable transmission, significant reduction in birth weight can be seen even in subsequent pregnancies (Nosten et al, 1991). Moreover, pregnant women in these areas tend to have more severe malarial infections (Looareesuwan et al, 1985). In vitro, there is impaired proliferative responses of peripheral and placental lymphocytes to malarial antigens (Rasheed et al, 1993), consistent with a general decrease in cellular immunity during pregnancy (Weinberg, 1984). On the other hand, anti-malarial antibody levels in pregnant women are comparable to those of controls.

The adverse effects of falciparum malaria on pregnancy have been variously attributed to the metabolic consequences of the infection (White et al, 1983), as well as to the immunosuppressive effects of increased corticosteroid and progesterone production (Vleugels et al, 1987; Szekeres-Bartho et al, 1990). The recent description of cytokine production at the maternal–fetal interface during pregnancy adds a further dimension to the host–parasite interaction (Wegmann et al, 1993). Th2 cytokines are produced during normal pregnancy, although the experimental results differ as to the predominance of IL-4 and IL-10 (Lin et al, 1993; Delassus et al, 1994). These cytokines are thought to be important for the maintenance of normal pregnancy by directing maternal immunity away from Th1 type cell-mediated responses which would lead to the elimination of the fetus. In this context, falciparum malaria infection during pregnancy can be seen to create a situation in which a shift in the Th1/Th2 balance may occur, with detrimental effects for both the mother and the fetus. Both IFN-γ and TNF-α have been shown to induce intrauterine growth retardation as well as spontaneous abortion in experimental models (Chaouat, 1994)

SUMMARY

The human immune response to the malaria parasite is complex, being determined by the large number of parasite antigens that are presented to the host, and the inability of most of the antigens to induce immunological memory. However, immunity can develop to all three stages of the parasite life cycle with repeated infections, although it is generally transient. Humoral immunity is important against sporozoites, asexual blood-stage parasites and gametocytes, either independently or in co-operation with effector cells such as mononuclear phagocytes and neutrophils. Antibody-independent cellular immunity has also been demonstrated against sporozoites in the form of cytotoxic CD8+ T cells; against asexual blood-stage parasites in the form of NK cells, γδ T cells and CD4+ and CD8+ αβ T cells; and against gametocytes in the form of TNF-α in the presence of as yet unidentified soluble mediators. While the spleen is crucial in anti-malarial immunity in experimental models, studies in human patients suggest that the function of the spleen may be assumed by other organs of the mononuclear phagocytic system. Disease manifestations are due almost exclusively to asexual blood-stage parasites through the process of cyto-adherence and the induction of TNF-α, IL-1 and IL-6. Parasite antigens also elicit intense T cell activation, resulting in markedly elevated levels of IFN-γ and IL-10. These cytokines have no direct role in immunopathology, but they are important in regulating the production of the inflammatory cytokines, and may partially explain the deleterious effect of malaria on both mother and fetus in pregnancy. Genetic restriction of responses to parasite antigens suggested by animal studies does not appear to be as important in outbred human populations, and although parasite antigens exhibit epitope polymorphism, the diversity is limited within a given geographical location. On the other hand, antigenic variation occurs spontaneously, and involves the cytoadherent ligand with resultant changes in receptor specificity. Aberrant immunological responses to malaria parasites are responsible for malarial nephropathy, Burkitt's lymphoma and hyper-reactive malarial splenomegaly.

Acknowledgements

The authors wish to thank the Medical Research Council of Canada, the Alberta Heritage Foundation for Medical Research, Canada, and the Wellcome-Mahidol University, Oxford Tropical Medicine Programme funded by the Wellcome Trust, UK for financial support, and Dr Nicholas J. White for valuable discussions and review of the manuscript.

REFERENCES

Abdurrahman MB, Aikhionbare HA, Babaoye FA, et al (1990) Clinicopathological features of childhood nephrotic syndrome in northern Nigeria. *Quarterly Journal of Medicine* **75:** 563–576.

Adebajo AO, Charles P, Maini RN & Hazleman BL (1993) Autoantibodies in malaria, tuberculosis and hepatitis B in a West African population. *Clinical and Experimental Immunology* **92:** 73–76.

Allen S, Van de Perre P, Serufilira A et al (1991) Human immunodeficiency virus and malaria in a representative sample of childbearing women in Kigali, Rwanda. *Journal of Infectious Diseases* **164:** 67–71.

Ballou WR, Hoffman SL, Sherwood JA et al (1987) Safety and efficacy of a recombinant DNA *Plasmodium falciparum* sporozoite vaccine. *Lancet* **i:** 1277–1281.

Bate CA & Kwiatkowski D (1994) Inhibitory immunoglobulin M antibodies to tumour necrosis factor-inducing toxins in patients with malaria. *Infection and Immunity* **62:** 3086–3091.

Bate CA, Taverne J, Roman E et al (1992) Tumour necrosis factor induction by malaria exoantigens depends upon phospholipid. *Immunology* **75:** 129–135.

Bate CA, Taverne J, Kwiatkowski D & Playfair JH (1993) Phospholipids coupled to a carrier induce IgG antibody that blocks tumour necrosis factor induction by toxic malaria antigens. *Immunology* **79:** 138–145.

Bates I, Bedu-Addo G, Bevan DH & Rutherford TR (1991) Use of immunoglobulin gene rearrangements to show clonal lymphoproliferation in hyper-reactive malarial splenomegaly. *Lancet* **337:** 505–507.

Biggs BA, Gooze L, Wycherley K et al (1991) Antigenic variation in *Plasmodium falciparum*. *Proceedings of the National Academy of Sciences of the USA* **88:** 9171–9174.

Boudin C, Dyannaz J, Rosseno MF et al (1991) Epidemiology of *Plasmodium falciparum* in a rice field and a savanna area in Burkina Faso: seasonal fluctuations of gametocytaemia and malarial infectivity. *Annals of Tropical Medicine and Parasitology* **85:** 377–385.

Bouharoun-Tayoun H & Druilhe P (1992) *Plasmodium falciparum* malaria: evidence for an isotype balance which may be responsible for delayed acquisition of protective immunity. *Infection and Immunity* **60:** 1473–1481.

Bouharoun-Tayoun H, Attanath P, Sabchareon A et al (1990) Antibodies that protect humans against *Plasmodium falciparum* blood stages do not on their own inhibit parasite growth and invasion in vitro, but act in cooperation with monocytes. *Journal of Experimental Medicine* **172:** 1633–1641.

Brabin BJ (1983) Analysis of malaria in pregnancy in Africa. *Bulletin of the World Health Organization* **61:** 1005–1016.

Bradley-Moore AM, Greenwood BM, Bradley AK et al (1985) Malaria chemoprophylaxis with chloroquine in young Nigerian children. 2. Effect on immune responses to vaccination. *Annals of Tropical Medicine and Parasitology* **79:** 563–573.

Brewster D, Kwiatkowski D & White NJ (1990) Neurological sequelae of cerebral malaria in childhood. *Lancet* **336:** 1039–1043.

Bruce-Chwatt LJ (1952) Malaria in African infants and children in southern Nigeria. *Annals of Tropical Medicine and Parasitology* **46:** 173–200.

Butcher GA (1992) HIV and malaria: a lesson in immunology? *Parasitology Today* **8:** 307–311.

Chaouat G (1994) Synergy of lipopolysaccharide and inflammatory cytokines in murine pregnancy: alloimmunization prevents abortion but does not affect the induction of preterm delivery. *Cellular Immunology* **157:** 328–340.

Clyde DF, Most H, McCarthy VC & Vanderberg JP (1973) Immunization of man against sporozoite-induced falciparum malaria. *American Journal of the Medical Sciences* **266:** 169–177.

Clyde DF, McCarthy VC, Miller RM & Woodward WE (1975) Immunization of man against falciparum and vivax malaria by use of attenuated sporozoites. *American Journal of Tropical Medicine and Hygiene* **24:** 397–401.

Cohen S, MacGregor IA & Carrington SC (1961) Gamma globulin and acquired immunity to human malaria. *Nature,* **192:** 733–737.

Daniel-Ribeiro C, Ben Slama L & Gentilin M (1991) Anti-nuclear and anti-smooth muscle antibodies in Caucasians, Africans and Asians with acute malaria. *Journal of Clinical and Laboratory Immunology* **35:** 109–112.

de Groot AS, Johnson AH, Maloy WL et al (1989) Human T cell recognition of polymorphic epitopes from malaria circumsporozoite protein. *Journal of Immunology* **142:** 4000–4005.

Delassus S, Coutinho GC, Saucier C et al (1994) Differential cytokine expression in maternal blood and placenta during murine gestation. *Journal of Immunology* **152:** 2411–2420.

Desowitz RS, Elm J & Alpers MP (1993) *Plasmodium*-specific immunoglobulin G (IgG), IgM, and IgE antibodies in paired maternal-cord sera from east Sepik Province, Papua New Guinea. *Infection and Immunity* **61:** 988–993.

Doolan D, Houghten RA & Good MF (1991) Location of human cytotoxic T cell epitopes within the polymorphic domain of the *Plasmodium falciparum* circumsporozoite protein. *International Immunology* **3:** 511–515.

Doolan DL, Saul AJ & Good MF (1992) Geographically restricted heterogeneity of the *Plasmodium falciparum* circumsporozoite protein: relevance for vaccine development. *Infection & Immunity* **60:** 675–682

Doolan DL, Khamboonruang C, Beck Hp et al (1993) Cytotoxic T lymphocyte low-responsiveness to the *Plasmodium falciparum* circumsporozoite protein in naturally exposed endemic populations: analysis of human CTL response to all known variants. *International Immunology* **5:** 37–46.

Doolan DL, Beck HP & Good MF (1994) Evidence for limited activation of distinct CD4+ T cell sub-sets in response to the *Plasmodium falciparum* circumsporozoite protein in Papua New Guinea. *Parasite Immunology* **16:** 129–136.

Elloso MM, van der Heyde HC, vande Waa JA et al (1994) Inhibition of *Plasmodium falciparum* in vitro by human δγT cells. *Journal of Immunology* **153:** 1187–1194.

Erunkulu OA, Hill AV, Kwiatkowski DP et al (1992) Severe malaria in Gambian children is not due to lack of previous exposure to malaria. *Clinical and Experimental Immunology* **89:** 296–300.

Fell AH, Currier J & Good MF (1994) Inhibition of *Plasmodium falciparum* growth in vitro by CD4⁺ and CD8⁺ T cells from non-exposed donors. *Parasite Immunology* **16:** 579–586.

Ferreira A, Schofield L, Enea V et al (1986) Inhibition of development of exoerythrocytic forms of malaria parasites by γ-interferon. *Science* **232:** 881–884.

Fleming AF (1990) Opportunistic infections in AIDS in developed and developing countries. *Transactions of the Royal Society of Tropical Medicine and Hygiene* **84 (supplement 1):** 1–6.

Fries LF, Gordon DM, Schneider I et al (1992) Safety, immunogenecity and efficacy of a *Plasmodium falciparum* vaccine comprising a circumsporozoite protein repeat region peptide conjugated to *Pseudomonas aeruginosa* toxin A. *Infection and Immunity* **60:** 1834–1839.

Gamage-Mendis AC, Rajakaruna J, Carter R & Mendis KN (1992) Transmission blocking immunity to human *Plasmodium vivax* malaria in an endemic population in Kataragama, Sri Lanka. *Parasite Immunology* **14:** 385–396.

Githeko AK, Brandling-Bennett AD, Beier M et al (1992) The reservoir of *Plasmodium falciparum* malaria in a holoendemic area of western Kenya. *Transactions of the Royal Society of Tropical Medicine and Hygiene* **86:** 355–358.

Good MF, Pombo D, Quakyi I et al (1988) Human T cell recognition of the circumsporozoite protein of *Plasmodium falciparum*. Immunodominant T cell domains map to the polymorphic regions of the molecule. *Proceedings of the National Academy of Sciences of the USA* **85:** 1119–1203.

Good MF, Kumar S, de Groot AS et al (1990) Evidence implicating MHC genes in the immunological nonresponsiveness to the *Plasmodium falciparum* CS protein. *Bulletin of the World Health Organization* **68 (supplement):** 80–84.

Good MF, Zevering Y, Currier J & Bilsborough J (1993) 'Original antigenic sin', T cell memory, and malaria sporozoite immunity: a hypothesis for immune evasion. *Parasite Immunology* **15:** 187–193.

Graves PM, Carter R, Burkot TR et al (1988) Antibodies to *Plasmodium falciparum* gamete surface antigens in Papua New Guinea sera. *Parasite Immunology* **10:** 209–218.

Grau GE, Taylor TE, Molyneux ME et al (1989) Tumour necrosis factor and disease severity in childen with falciparum malaria. *New England Journal of Medicine* **320:** 1586–1591.

Greenberg AE, Nsa W, Ryder RW et al (1991) *Plasmodium falciparum* malaria and perinatally acquired human immunodeficiency virus type I infection in Kinshasa Zaire. *New England Journal of Medicine* **325:** 105–109.

Greenwood BM, Bradley-Moore AM, Palit A & Bryceson ADM (1972) Immunosuppression in children with malaria. *Lancet* **i:** 169–172.

Greenwood BM, Bradley AK, Greenwood AM et al (1987) Mortality and morbidity from malaria among children in a rural area of The Gambia, West Africa. *Transactions of the Royal Society of Tropical Medicine and Hygiene* **81:** 478–486.

Grun JL & Weidanz WP (1981) Immunity to *Plasmodium chabaudi adami* in the B-cell deficient mouse. *Nature* **290:** 143–145.

Handunnetti SM, Mendis KN & David PH (1987) Antigenic variation of cloned *P. fragile* in its natural host *Macaca sinica*. Sequential appearance of successive variant antigenic types. *Journal of Experimental Medicine* **165:** 1269–1283.

Hendrickse RG, Adeniyi A, Edington GM et al (1977) Quartan malarial nephrotic syndrome. Collaborative clinicopathological study in Nigerian children. *Lancet* **i:** 1143–1149.

Herrington DA, Clyde DF, Losonsky G et al (1987) Safety and immunogenicity in man of a synthetic peptide tetanus toxoid conjugate malaria vaccine against *Plasmodium falciparum* sporozoites. *Nature* **328:** 257–259.

Hill AVS, Allsopp CEM, Kwiatkowski D et al (1991) Common West African HLA antigens are associated with protection from severe malaria. *Nature* **352:** 595–600.

Ho M & Webster HK (1990) T cell responses in acute falciparum malaria. *Immunology Letters* **25:** 135–138.

Ho M, Webster, HK, Looareesuwan S et al (1986) Antigen-specific immunosuppression in human malaria due to *Plasmodium falciparum*. *Journal of Infectious Diseases* **153:** 763–771.

Ho M, Webster HK, Green B et al (1988) Defective production of and response to interleukin 2 in acute falciparum malaria. *Journal of Immunology* **141:** 2755–2759.

Ho M, White NJ, Looareesuwan S et al (1991) Splenic Fc receptor function in host defense and anemia in acute *Plasmodium falciparum* malaria. *Journal of Infectious Diseases* **161:** 555–561.

Ho M, Tongtawe P, Kriangkum J et al (1994) Polyclonal expansion of peripheral T cells in human *Plasmodium falciparum* malaria. *Infection and Immunity* **62:** 855–861.

Ho M, Sexton MM, Tongtawe P et al (in press) Interleukin-10 inhibits tumor necrosis factor production but not antigen-specific lymphoproliferation in acute *Plasmodium falciparum* malaria. *Journal of Infectious Diseases*.

Hoffman SL, Piessens WF, Ratiwayanto S et al (1984) Reduction of suppressor T lymphocytes in the tropical splenomegaly syndrome. *New England Journal of Medicine* **310:** 337–341.

Hoffman SL, Oster CN, Mason C et al (1989) Human lymphocyte proliferative response to a sporo-zoite T cell epitope correlates with resistance to falciparum malaria. *Journal of Immunology* **142:** 1299–1303.

Hollingdale MR, Nardin EH, Tharavanij S et al (1984) Inhibition of entry of *Plasmodium falciparum* and *Plasmodium vivax* sporozoites into cultured cells, an in vitro assay of protective antibodies. *Journal of Immunology* **132:** 909–913.

Imberti L, Sottini A, Bettinardi A et al (1991) Selective depletion in HIV infection of T cells that bear specific T cell receptor V β sequences. *Science* **254:** 860–862.

Jakobsen PH, Morris-Jones S, Theander TG et al (1994) Increased plasma levels of soluble IL-2R are associated with severe *Plasmodium falciparum* malaria. *Clinical Experimental Immunology* **96:** 98–108.

Kabelitz D, Bender A, Schondelmaier S et al (1990) A large fraction of human peripheral blood γ/δ+ T cells is activated by *Mycobacterium tuberculosis* but not by its 65-kd heat shock protein. *Journal of Experimental Medicine* **171:** 667–679.

Karunaweera ND, Carter R, Grau GE et al (1993) Tumour necrosis factor-dependent parasite-killing effects during paroxysms in non-immune *Plasmodium vivax* malaria patients. *Clinical Experimental Immunology* **88:** 499–505.

Kumaratilake LM & Ferrante A (1992) IL-4 inhibits macrophage-mediated killing of *Plasmodium falciparum* in vitro. A possible parasite-immune evasion mechanism. *Journal of Immunology* **149:** 194–199.

Kumaratilake LM, Ferrante A & Rzepczyk C (1991) The role of T lymphocytes in immunity to *Plasmodium falciparum*. Enhancement of neutrophil-mediated parasite killing by lymphotoxin and IFN-γ comparisons with tumour necrosis factor effects. *Journal of Immunology* **146:** 762–767.

Kumaratilake LM, Ferrante A, Jaeger T & Rzepczyk CM (1992) Effects of cytokines, complement, and antibody on the neutrophil respiratory burst and phagocytic response to *Plasmodium falciparum* merozoites. *Infection and Immunity* **60:** 3731–3738.

Kwiatkowski D, Hill AVS, Sambou I et al (1990) TNF concentrations in fatal cerebral, non-fatal cerebral, and uncomplicated *Plasmodium falciparum* malaria. *Lancet* **336:** 1021–1024.

Lam KMC, Syed N, Whittle H & Crawford D (1991) Circulating Epstein–Barr virus-carrying B cells in acute malaria. *Lancet* **337:** 876–878.

Lin H, Mosmann TR, Guilbert L et al (1993) Synthesis of T helper 2-type cytokines at the maternal-fetal interface. *Journal of Immunology* **151:** 4562–4573.

Looareesuwan S, Phillips RE, White NJ et al (1985) Quinine and severe malaria in late pregnancy. *Lancet* **ii:** 4–8.

Looareesuwan S, Ho M, Wattanagoon Y et al (1987a) Dynamic alteration in splenic function during acute falciparum malaria. *New England Journal of Medicine* **317:** 675–679.

Looareesuwan S, Merry AH, Phillips RE et al (1987b) Reduced erythrocyte survival following clear-ance of malarial parasitaemia in Thai patients. *British Journal of Haematology* **67:** 473–478.

Looareesuwan S, Suntharasamai P, Webster HK & Ho M (1993) Malaria in splenectomized patients: report of four cases and review. *Clinical Infectious Diseases* **16:** 361–366.

Magrath I, Jain V & Bhatia K (1992) Epstein–Barr virus and Burkitt's Lymphoma. *Seminars in Cancer Biology* **3:** 285–295.

Marsh K & Greenwood BM (1986) The immunopathology of malaria. *Clinics in Tropical Medicine And Communicable Diseases* **1:** 91–126.

Marsh K & Howard RJ (1986) Antigens induced on erythrocytes by *P. falciparum:* expression of diverse and conserved determinants. *Science* **231:** 150–153.

Masucci MG & Klein E (1991) Cell phenotype dependent expression of MHC class 1 antigens in Burkitt's lymphoma cell lines. *Seminars in Cancer Biology* **2:** 63–71.

McGregor IA (1984) Epidemiology, malaria and pregnancy. *American Journal of Tropical Medicine and Hygiene* **33:** 517–525.

Mendis KN, Munesinghe YD, de Silva YN et al (1987) Malaria transmission-blocking immunity induced by natural infections of *Plasmodium vivax* in humans. *Infections and Immunity* **55:** 369–372.

Mendis KN, Ihalamulla RI & David PH (1988) Diversity of *Plasmodium vivax*-induced antigens on the surface of infected human erythrocytes. *American Journal of Tropical Medicine and Hygiene* **38:** 40–42.

Muller O & Moser R (1990) The clinical and parasitological presentation of *Plasmodium falciparum* malaria in Uganda is unaffected by HIV-1 infection. *Transactions of the Royal Society of Tropical Medicine and Hygiene* **84:** 336–338.

Murray HW & Teitelbaum RF (1992) L-arginine-dependent reactive nitrogen intermediates and the antimicrobial effect of activated human mononuclear phagocytes. *Journal of Infectious Diseases* **165:** 513–517.

Naotunne TS, Karunaweera ND, Mendis KN & Carter R (1993) Cytokine-mediated inactivation of malarial gametocytes is dependent on the presence of white blood cells and involves reactive nitrogen intermediates. *Immunology* **78:** 555–562.

Niyongabo T, Deloran P, Aubry P et al (1994) Prognostic indicators in adult cerebral malaria: a study in Burundi, an area of high prevalence of HIV infection. *Acta Tropica* **56:** 299–305.

Nosten F, ter Kuile F, Malankiri L et al (1991) Malaria in pregnancy in an area of unstable endemicity. *Transactions of the Royal Society of Tropical Medicine and Hygiene* **85:** 424–429.

Ockenhouse CF, Magowan C & Chulay JD (1989) Activation of monocytes and platelets by monoclonal antibodies or malaria-infected erythrocytes binding to the CD36 surface receptor in vitro. *Journal of Clinical Investigations* **84:** 468–475.

Oppenheimer SJ, Macfarlane SBJ, Moody JB et al (1986) Effect of iron prophylaxis on morbidity due to infectious diseases: report on clinical studies in Papua New Guinea. *Transactions of the Royal Society of Tropical Medicine and Hygiene* **80:** 603–612.

Orago ASS & Facer CA (1991) Cytotoxicity of human natural killer (NK) cell subsets for *Plasmodium falciparum* erythrocyte schizonts: stimulation by cytokines and inhibition by neomycin. *Clinical and Experimental Immunology* **86:** 23–29.

Pasvol G, Weatherall DJ, Wilson RJM et al (1976) Foetal haemoglobin and malaria. *Lancet* **i:** 1269–1272.

Perera MK, Carter R, Goonewardene R & Mendis KN (1994) Transient increase in circulating gamma/delta T cells during *Plasmodium vivax* malarial paroxysms. *Journal of Experimental Medicine* **179:** 311–315.

Peyron F, Burdin N, Ringwald P et al (1994) High levels of circulating IL-10 in human malaria. *Clinical and Experimental Immunology* **95:** 300–306.

Phanuphak P, Hanvanich M, Sakulramrung R et al (1985) Complement changes in falciparum malaria infection. *Clinical and Experimental Immunology* **59:** 571–576.

Picot S, Peyron F, Vuillez JP et al (1990) Tumour necrosis factor production by human macrophages stimulated in vitro by *Plasmodium falciparum*. *Infection and Immunity* **58:** 214–216.

Picot S, Peyron F, Deloron P et al (1993) Ring-infected erythrocyte surface antigen (Pf/155RESA) induces tumour necrosis factor-α production. *Clinical Experimental Immunology* **93:** 184–188.

Pied S, Renia L, Nussier et al (1991) Inhibitory activity of IL-6 on malaria hepatic stages. *Parasite Immunology* **13:** 211–217.

Piessens WF, Hoffman SL Wadee AA et al (1985) Antibody mediated killing of T suppressor lymphocytes as a possible cause of macroglobulinemia in the tropical splenomegaly syndrome. *Journal of Clinical Investigations* **75:** 1821–1827.

Playfair JHL, Taverne J, Bate CAW & de Souza JB (1990) The malaria vaccine: anti-parasite or anti-disease? *Immunology Today* **11:** 25–27.

Pongpanratn E, Riganti M, Harinasuta T & Bunnag D (1989) Electron microscopic study of phagocytosis in human spleen in falciparum malaria. *Southeast Asian Journal of Tropical Medicine and Public Health* **20:** 31–39.

Porcelli S, Brenner MB & Band H (1991) Biology of the human γδ T-cell receptor. *Immunological Review* **120:** 137–183.

Qari SH, Goldman IF, Pavoa MM et al (1992) Polymorphism in the circumsporozoite protein of the human malaria parasite *Plasmodium vivax*. *Molecular and Biochemical Parasitology* **55:** 105–113.

Quakyi IA, Otoo LN, Pombo D et al (1989) Differential non-responsiveness in humans of candidate *Plasmodium falciparum* vaccine antigens. *American Journal of Tropical Medicine and Hygiene* **41:** 125–134.

Rasheed FN, Bukmer JN, Dunn DT et al (1993) Suppressed peripheral and placental blood lymphoproliferative responses in first pregnancies: relevance to malaria. *American Journal of Tropical Medicine and Hygiene* **48:** 154–160.

Riley EM (1994) Regulation of the immune response to malaria: selective recognition of malaria antigens by human serum antibodies. *XIII International Congress of Parasitology*, 10–14 October, Izmir Turkey (abstract no. 677).

Riley E & Greenwood B (1990) Measuring cellular immune response to malaria antigens in endemic populations: epidemiological, parasitological and physiological factors which influence in vitro assays. *Immunology Letters* **25:** 221–229.

Riley EM, MacLennan C, Kwiatkowski DK & Greenwood BM (1989) Suppression of in vitro lymphoproliferative response in acute malaria patients can be partially reversed by indomethacin. *Parasite Immunology* **11**: 509–517.

Riley EM, Allen SJ, Bennett S et al (1990) Recognition of dominant T cell-stimulating epitopes from the circumsporozoite protein of *Plasmodium falciparum* and relationship to malaria morbidity in Gambian children. *Transactions of the Royal Society of Tropical Medicine and Hygiene* **84**: 648–657.

Riley EM, Olerup O, Bennett S et al (1992) MHC and malaria: the relationship between HLA class II alleles and immune responses to *Plasmodium falciparum*. *International Immunology* **4**: 1055–1063.

Ritter K, Kuhlencord A, Thomssen R & Bommer W (1993) Prolonged haemolytic anaemia in malaria and autoantibodies against triosephosphate isomerase. *Lancet* **342**: 1333–1334.

Roberts DJ, Craig AG, Berendt AR et al (1992) Rapid switching to multiple antigenic and adhesive phenotypes in malaria. *Nature* **357**: 689–692.

Rockett AK, Awburn MM, Cowden WB & Clark IA (1991) Killing of *Plasmodium falciparum* in vitro by nitric oxide derivatives. *Infection and Immunity* **59**: 3280–3283.

Roussilhon C, Agarapart M, Guglielmi P et al (1994) Human TcR+ lymphocyte response on primary exposure to *Plasmodium falciparum*. *Clinical and Experimental Immunology* **95**: 91–97.

Sabchareon A, Rurnouf T, Ouattara D et al (1991) Parasitological and clinical human response to immunoglobulin administration in falciparum malaria. *American Journal of Tropical Medicine and Hygiene* **45**: 297–308.

Schwarzer E, Turrini F, Ulliers D et al (1992) Impairment of macrophage functions after ingestion of *Plasmodium falciparum*-infected erythrocytes or isolated malarial pigment. *Journal of Experimental Medicine* **176**: 1033–1041.

Sedegah M, Sim BKL, Mason et al (1992) Naturally acquired CD8+ cytotoxic T lymphocytes against the *Plasmodium falciparum* circumsporozoite protein. *Journal of Immunology* **149**: 966–971.

Serjeantson SW & Crane GG (1991) Analysis of the patterns of inheritance of splenomegaly and serum IgG levels in the Watut of Papua New Guinea. *Human Biology* **63**: 115–128.

Sinton JA, Harbhagwan M & Singh J (1931) The numerical prevalence of parasites in relation to fever in chronic benign tertian malaria. *Indian Journal of Medical Research* **18**: 871–874.

Snow RW, Bastps de Azevedo I, Lowe BS et al (1994) Severe childhood malaria in two areas of markedly different *P. falciparum* transmission in East Africa. *Acta Tropica* **57**: 289–300.

Szekeres–Bartho J, Philibert D & Chaouat G (1990) Progesterone suppression of pregnancy lymphocytes is not mediated by glucocorticoid effect. *American Journal of Reproductive Immunology* **23**: 42–43.

Troye–Blomberg M, Romero M, Patarroya ME et al (1984) Regulation of the immune responses in *Plasmodium falciparum* malaria. II. Proliferative response to antigen in vitro and subset composition of T cells from patients with acute infection or from immune donors. *Clinical Experimental Immunology* **58**: 380–387.

van der Heyde HC, Huszar D, Woodhouse C et al (1994) The resolution of acute malaria in a definitive model of B cell deficiency, the JHD mouse. *Journal of Immunology* **152**: 4557–4562.

Vleugels MPH, Eling WMC, Rolland R & De Graaf R (1987) Cortisol and loss of malaria immunity in human pregnancy. *British Journal of Obstetrics and Gynaecology* **94**: 758–764.

Webster HK, Ho M, Looareesuwan S et al (1989) Lymphocyte responsiveness to a candidate malaria sporozoite vaccine (R32$_{tet32}$) of individuals with naturally acquired *Plasmodium falciparum* malaria. *American Journal of Tropical Medicine and Hygiene* **38**: 37–41.

Wegmann T, Lin H, Guilbert L & Mosmann T (1993) Bidirectional cytokine interactions in the maternal-fetal relationship: is successful pregnancy a Th2 phenomenon? *Immunology Today* **14**: 353–356.

Weinberg ED (1984) Pregnancy-associated depression of cell-mediated immunity. *Review of Infectious Diseases* **6**: 814–831.

Weiss L, Geduldig U & Weidanz WP (1986) Mechanisms of splenic control murine malaria: reticular cell activation and the development of a blood-spleen barrier. *American Journal of Anatomy* **176**: 251–285.

Weiss WR, Melleuk S, Houghton RA et al (1990) Cytotoxic T cells recognize a peptide from the circumsporozoite protein on malaria-infected hepatocytes. *Journal of Experimental Medicine* **171**: 763–773.

White NJ, Warrell DA, Looareesuwan S et al (1983) Hypoglycaemia and hyperinsulinaemia in falciparum malaria. *New England Journal of Medicine* **309**: 61–66.

Whittle HC, Brown J, Marsh K et al (1984) T-cell contro of Epstein–Barr virus-infected B cells is lost during *P. falciparum* malaria. *Nature* **312**: 449–450.

Wongsrichanalai C, Webster, HK, Permpanich B et al (1991) Naturally acquired circumsporozoite antibodies and their role in protection in endemic falciparum and vivax malaria. *American Journal of Tropical Medicine and Hygiene* **44**: 201–204.

Wyler DJ, Oster CN & Quinn TC (1983) The role of the spleen in malaria infections. In *UNDP/World Bank/WHO Special Programme for Research and Training in Tropical Diseases. Role of the Spleen in the Immunology of Parasitic Diseases*, pp 183–204. Basel: Schwabe & Co.

Yoshida N, Di Santi SM, Dutra AP et al (1990) *Plasmodium falciparum*: restricted polymorphism of T cell epitopes of the circumsporozoite protein in Brazil. *Experimental Parasitology* **71**: 386–392.

Zevering Y, Amante F, Smillie A et al (1992) High frequency of malaria-specific T cells in non-exposed humans. *European Journal of Immunology* **22**: 689–696.

Zevering Y, Khamboonruang C, Rungruengthanakit K et al (1994) Life-spans of human T-cell responses to determinants from the circumsporozoite proteins of *Plasmodium falciparum* and *Plasmodium vivax*. *Proceedings of the National Academy of Sciences of the USA* **91**: 6118–6122.

3

The pathogenesis of severe falciparum malaria

GEOFFREY PASVOL
BARBARA CLOUGH
JAN CARLSSON
GEORGES SNOUNOU

Malaria is a disease to which over one quarter of the world's population remains at risk and in whom there are up to 250 million clinical cases annually. Of the four species of malaria parasites known to infect man, *Plasmodium vivax, P. ovale* and *P. malariae* undoubtedly cause major morbidity, but result in little mortality. *Plasmodium falciparum*, by contrast, is responsible for over one million deaths in Africa each year (Sturchler, 1989). One of the central outstanding questions in malaria is 'Why do patients with severe disease due to *P. falciparum* become so sick and die?' This chapter aims to elaborate on some of the factors involved, and to provide an answer, albeit incomplete, to this seemingly simple question.

At any one time many of the population living in an endemic area are infected with malaria parasites but remain asymptomatic. Only a minority develop symptomatic disease and even fewer progress to combinations of the three major manifestations of severe disease, namely, anaemia, cerebral malaria and respiratory distress (Marsh et al, 1995). Why individuals, especially children, should progress from being infected and asymptomatic, to being symptomatic with mild disease or develop fulminating disease and sometimes die, is poorly understood (Greenwood et al, 1991). The relative incidence of the many complications of malaria vary, perhaps depending on endemicity and age. In Africa, compared with South East Asia for example, renal failure, pulmonary oedema, circulatory collapse and disseminated intravascular coagulation are rare. In holoendemic (continuous sustained exposure) areas anaemia tends to dominate, whereas in hyperendemic (seasonal exposure) areas there is a relative increase in cerebral cases. In Africa, the peak age prevalence of malarial anaemia clearly precedes that of cerebral malaria but this is not due to lack of exposure to the parasite by those individuals developing cerebral manifestations, i.e. children developing cerebral malaria are not encountering the parasite for the first time (Erunkulu et al, 1992).

The pathogenesis of malaria is clearly the result of complex interactions between the parasite, the host and the environment (Table 1). However, in malaria it is important to realize that the 'unit of pathology' is the infected

Baillière's Clinical Infectious Diseases —
Vol. 2, No. 2, July 1995
ISBN 0–7020–1983–6

249

red cell, the properties of which are a combination of both host and parasite. Interactions between parasite and host such as the invasion of uninfected red cells, cytoadherence, rosetting and recognition of infected cells by macrophages, are interactions reflecting both parasite and host determinants (Pasvol et al, 1992). Two excellent and detailed reviews on the pathophysiology can be found elsewhere (Warrell et al, 1990; White, 1992).

Table 1. Factors associated with severe falciparum malaria in man.
'Why do patients with falciparum malaria become so sick and die?'

In severe malaria no consistent
  Inflammatory infiltrate
  Tissue death
  Breakdown of the blood–brain barrier
  Cerebral oedema
  Disseminated intravascular coagulation
  Hypoglycaemia

Parasite–host interactions
  No specific parasite genotype identified as yet
  Possible phenotypic associations
    Invasion
    Cytoadherence
    Rosetting
    Toxin production
    Others

Host
  Innate:
  Red cell variants – haemoglobin, membrane, enzymes
  MHC class I and II
  TNF-α promoter region
  Others, e.g. acidglycoprotein

  Acquired:
  Immunity
  Age
  Pregnancy
  Superinfection
  Mixed malarial infection
  Nutrition

  Environment:
  Absence or failure of prophylaxis
  Delay in treatment
  Failure of compliance with prophylaxis
  Iatrogenic

PARASITE–HOST INTERACTIONS

A number of cellular and molecular interactions occurring between the human host and the parasite stand out in the pathogenesis of severe malaria. These include the degree to which red cells are invaded by merozoites, the adherence of schizont-infected red cells to endothelial cells, the rosetting of uninfected red cells around schizont-infected red cells and the production of a 'toxin' or 'toxins' by the parasitized red cell leading to the release of numerous cytokines, of which tumour necrosis factor-α (TNF-α) and interleukin 1 (IL-1) appear to occupy a central role (Clark et al, 1989). One of the goals of parasite biology research has been to identify parasite phenotypes and/or genotypes conferring parasite virulence. Unfortunately this goal remains unfulfilled at present.

Parasite multiplication and invasion

It would appear that within a given individual, severity of malarial disease relates to parasite density, which in turn relates to the ability of the parasite to multiply, not only within the liver but, perhaps more importantly, within red cells. However, care must be taken on two counts when relating parasite density in peripheral blood to disease severity. First, tolerance to a given parasite burden differs between hosts because of both innate and acquired factors (see below). Second, sequestration of parasites in the deep tissues could result in a gross underestimation of the total parasite load as judged by peripheral parasite counts. Moreover factors operating at a stage earlier than multiplication within the liver or red cells could also be involved in the expression of pathology, and so the issue of infecting dose and disease severity remains an unresolved one. A direct relationship has been found recently between the degree of exposure of individuals to infected mosquitoes in the previous 28 days and parasite density in the peripheral blood (McElroy et al, 1994). Whether these observations could be explained by an increase in the number of sporozoites injected, by an increase in the diversity of infecting parasites, or both, remains to be established. Nonetheless, such an observation has major relevance, since previous thinking had assumed that limitation of the number of sporozoites reaching the liver or the number of merozoites released from the liver, would not reduce morbidity or mortality.

Invasion of red cells

Paramount to our understanding of the pathogenesis of malaria is that the parasite invades only red cells (and occasionally platelets), a property shared by very few parasites in man other than *Bartonella bacilliformis* and *Babesia spp.*, and that the rate and degree to which the parasite multiplies in some way relates to disease severity. In turn, the ability of *P. falciparum* to invade cells of all ages in contrast to, say, the reticulocyte restriction of *P. vivax*, enhances its multiplicative ability although even *P. falciparum* maintains a predilection for younger red cells (Pasvol et al, 1980).

Invasion is a highly specific, ordered and sequential process in which the merozoite attaches to a susceptible red cell, reorientates itself so that its apical end is apposed to the red cell membrane, and then slowly moves into a localized invagination of the red cell (Pasvol et al, 1993; Ward et al, 1994). The entire process of invasion is completed within 30 seconds. Identification of the molecules on the red cell surface to which the merozoites bind has recently been the subject of intense research. The red cell sialoglycoproteins or glycophorins (GPs), especially GPA and GPB, play a major role (Pasvol, 1984). In the search for a merozoite-binding site on GPA one particular epitope, Wr[b], appeared particularly interesting, as a number of anti-Wr[b] monoclonal antibodies markedly inhibited invasion (Pasvol et al, 1982). However, when Wr[b] negative cells were tested, they were fully susceptible to invasion indicating that the antibodies were acting via mechanisms other than receptor blockade. Of the sites involved on GPs, the O-linked tetrasaccharides, rather than the very much larger N-linked sugars on these molecules, were found to be relevant (Pasvol et al, 1987). Invasion by parasites of uninfected cells appears to correlate with the binding of a conserved parasite molecule, the erythrocyte binding antigen of molecular mass 175 kDa (EBA 175), to these cells (Sim et al, 1990). EBA 175 appears to recognize N-acetylneuraminic (sialic) acid linked in an α 2-3 configuration to galactose, but not the other sialic acid of the tetrasaccharide on the GP, linked in an α 2-6 configuration to N-acetylgalactosamine (Orlandi et al, 1992). A cleavage product of EBA 175, having a molecular mass of 65 kDa, which subsequently binds to red cells appears not to require sialic acid (Kain et al, 1993). However, there are also $P.$ $falciparum$ parasites capable of invading cells devoid of GPA or GPB (Hadley et al, 1987), which, if not sialic acid independent, are less sialic acid dependent in their invasion requirements. Such a change in invasion requirements may involve a switching mechanism (Dolan et al, 1990). Current evidence does not indicate a role for red cell band 3 (the major anion transporter) in merozoite recognition of red cells, although band 3 may be involved in subsequent steps in the invasion process.

Once attachment and orientation have occurred, interiorization accompanied by deformation of the red cell membrane follows, but the molecules involved in this part of the process have not as yet been identified. Testing red cell deformability by ektacytometry (which examines how cells deform when exposed to shear stress), and lateral mobility of transmembrane proteins, GPs and band 3 using the method of fluorescence recovery after photobleaching (FRAP), indicate that alterations in the physicochemical properties of the red cell membrane might well be responsible for the observed decreased invasion induced by antibodies to the red cell (e.g. anti-Wr[b]) and other red cell ligands (Pasvol et al, 1989; Clough et al, 1995).

Identification of the parasite components, in contrast to the red cell components involved in invasion, is even more complex and at least nine different parasite proteins of $P.$ $falciparum$ located on a variety of microorganelles of the parasite have been implicated in invasion (Perkins, 1991). The better known of these include the merozoite surface protein-1 having a molecular mass of 195 kDa (MSP-1) and the apical membrane antigen-1 (AMA-1) again found in the merozoite. For a detailed description and review of the host and parasite molecules involved in invasion see Ward et al (1994).

Whilst the multiplicative ability of the asexual form of $P.$ $falciparum$ is clearly variable in vitro, technical difficulties and the process of sequestration have made the question of whether enhanced invasion by parasites constitutes a virulence factor in vivo, difficult to answer. Schizonts of *P. falciparum* have a theoretical multiplicative potential of between 16 and 32, each possessing this number of merozoites on average, but such a degree of multiplication has not been documented in vivo or in vitro. Rather, a figure of between three- and ten-fold obtains (White et al, 1992).

When the phenomenon of rosetting was first observed (see below), it was argued that rosette formation, by juxtaposing infected and uninfected cells, might function as a major 'virulence' factor. Rosetting, it was argued, would enhance invasion and parasite multiplication especially under conditions of flow as occurs in the microvasculature of the deep tissues where invasion is thought to occur. However, rigorous experiments with a rosetting and non-rosetting parasite line, under static conditions or with red cells maintained under conditions of flow, have demonstrated that rosetting neither increases invasion, nor does it target parasites within a rosette at abutting uninfected cells (B. Clough et al, unpublished data).

Cytoadherence

Cytoadherence is the process whereby mature infected cells specifically bind to endothelial cells in post-capillary venules (Udeinya et al, 1981), and appears to play a central role in the pathogenesis of *P. falciparum* malaria (Berendt et al, 1990). If examined by scanning electron microscopy, a number of regular, symmetrically arranged 'knobs' appear on the surface of the cell as the immature parasite of *P. falciparum* develops. These knobs are thought to be the site at which the parasitized red cell attaches to the endothelial cell in the deep tissues, although parasites without knobs are capable of cytoadherence in vitro. Several proteins occurring in association with the knobs have been identified and include:

(i)   The histidine rich protein (HRP-I) which induces an excrescence below the bilipid layer of the red cell and which is thought to be attached to the red cell cytoskeleton. Interestingly a monoclonal antibody to HRP-I can disrupt rosettes (Carlson et al, 1990b).

(ii) A number of high molecular weight proteins which are thought to protrude from the knob of which the best known is the *P. falciparum* erythrocyte membrane protein 1 (Pf EMP-1). This molecule shows variation in size and antigenic properties.

(iii) A knob-associated structural protein, mature-parasite-infected erythrocyte surface antigen (MESA), also known as Pf EMP-2.

(iv) A modification of the major red cell anion transporter, band 3, has also been implicated as having a major role in cytoadherence (Winograd and Sherman, 1989).

Pf EMP-1 undergoes phenotypic antigenic variation, analogous in many ways to the variable coat of the trypanosome which is shed under immune pressure to be replaced by a different variant. Such a mechanism may be responsible, at least in part, for host immune evasion. Purification of Pf

EMP-1 has been elusive, although adult hyperimmune sera can precipitate this antigen, which seems to be exclusively located at the site of the knob. Pf EMP-1 may bind to a number of potential ligands on the surface of endothelial cells which at present include:

(i)   The adhesion molecule CD36 expressed on platelets, monocytes/ macrophages, early red cell precursors and at low level on endothelial cells (Udeinya et al, 1981).

(ii) Thrombospondin, a major component of the platelet-α granule (Roberts et al, 1985).

(iii) Two members of the immunoglobulin (Ig) superfamily, intercellular adhesion molecule 1 (ICAM-1) the ligand for the leukocyte integrin lymphocyte function-related antigen (LFA-1) (Berendt et al, 1989), and vascular cell adhesion molecule (VCAM-1) (Ockenhouse et al, 1992).

(iv) E-selectin (Ockenhouse et al, 1992).

However, the specificity of binding to each of these various molecules is thought to be quite different, and it has yet to be established which of these ligands is/are the definitive receptor(s) for the binding of parasitized cells in man. Whether Pf EMP-1 is the molecule that binds to all has yet to be established. ICAM-1, VCAM-1 and E-selectin, but not CD36 and thrombo-spondin, are upregulated by cytokines (Esslinger et al, 1994). In malaria, ICAM-1 appears to act as a rolling receptor, whereas CD36 and thrombo-spondin seem to be involved in more stable interactions (Cooke et al, 1994). Higher levels of ICAM-1 and E-selectin were detected by immuno-chemistry on vessels in the brain of patients with severe malaria compared to uninfected controls, whereas endothelial CD36 and thrombospondin showed no increase (Turner et al, 1995). At the sites of sequestration there was co-localization of ICAM-1, CD36 and thrombospondin but no evidence of a cellular inflammatory response.

Whatever the specific mechanisms for cytoadherence, a more pertinent question is the significance of cytoadherence in pathogenesis. Cyto-adherence by immobilizing parasites in various organs will prevent their passage through the spleen, a major site of parasite destruction; will local-ize maturing parasites at sites of reduced oxygen tension which favours parasite growth; and may facilitate invasion of uninfected red cells. In the process of cytoadherence, parasites may produce damage in a number of ways, although several studies have failed to find an association between cytoadherence and severe disease (Marsh et al, 1988; Goldring et al, 1992). Cytoadherent parasites presumably lead to microvascular obstruction, although the role and extent of this obstruction remains unclear (Wick and Louis, 1991). Total cerebral blood flow in cerebral malaria remains un-altered and tissue infarction and necrosis, an expected sequel of micro-circulatory blockage, is uncommon. Cytoadherence may lead to endothelial cell activation and/or damage, release of cytokines by these cells and in particular may serve to concentrate the release of parasite toxins and sub-stances induced by such toxins locally (See Chapter 9: The biology of malarial fever).

Rosetting

In rosetting, an interaction quite distinct from cytoadherence, red cells containing the more mature stages of the parasite bind uninfected red cells to their surface (David et al, 1988; Handunnetti et al, 1989; Udomsangpetch et al, 1989). Interest in rosetting derives from its possible role as a parasite virulence factor. In studies in The Gambia, all isolates of *P. falciparum* obtained from children with cerebral malaria were capable of rosetting, whereas many isolates from patients with mild disease were not (Carlson et al, 1990a; Ringwald et al, 1993). Moreover, plasma from children with mild disease could more often disrupt preformed rosettes than plasma from patients with cerebral malaria. The anti-rosetting activity was present in the immunoglobulin fraction. However, not all studies are in agreement (Hasler et al, 1990; Ho et al, 1991).

A monoclonal antibody to HRP-I has been shown to specifically disrupt rosettes, a surprising finding since the location of this protein is below the bilipid layer of the red cell within the cytoskeleton (Carlson et al, 1990b). This phenomenon can however be explained by cross-reactivity of these antibodies with low molecular mass molecules thought to be on the surface of the infected red cell (the 'rosettins': Helmby et al, 1993). However, the definitive molecular components of rosetting on the infected and uninfected red cell have yet to be resolved. Whilst one group has implicated the rosettins on the infected cell and the ABO blood group sugar molecules on the uninfected cell (especially A or B) (Carlson and Wahlgren, 1992), another group has implicated Pf EMP-1 and CD36, respectively (Handunnetti et al, 1992).

The mechanisms by which rosetting leads to disease remain obscure, although it is the only parasite phenotype to date that has shown a clear association with cerebral malaria. Rosetting parasites when perfused in an ex vivo model of the rat mesoappendix, result in greater vascular resistance when compared to non-rosetting parasites (Kaul et al, 1991). Rosetting, as mentioned above, does not appear to enhance merozoite invasion (B. Clough et al, unpublished data). It also remains possible that parasites within the protective barrier of a rosette are less easily the target of (antibody-mediated) macrophage recognition and removal. Such a mechanism may well turn out to be the major mechanism of immunity in malaria infection (Bouharoun et al, 1990).

Toxins and cytokines

Attempts to identify a definitive malarial toxin remain unresolved. The glycosylphosphatidylinositol (GPI)-anchored molecules of the parasite are favoured candidates (Schofield and Hackett, 1993; Gerold et al, 1994), but other molecules have been proposed, including as yet undefined phospholipid molecules (Bate et al, 1992) and a protease-sensitive component of malarial pigment (Pichyangkul et al, 1994: see Chapter 9). Even products from lysed uninfected red cells are capable of inducing cytokine release, although at least 200 times less so than parasitized cells (Bate and

Kwiatkowski, 1994). The concept of a malarial toxin becomes important as there is re-emerging evidence of an age-old belief that malaria is a 'metabolic' disorder, perturbing many aspects of the immune system including the cytokines and their receptors.

Whatever the case, it is proposed that such a toxin or toxins result(s) in the release, amongst others, of the cytokines TNF and IL-1 (Clark et al, 1989; Harpaz et al, 1992; Grau and de Kossodo, 1994). There is certainly a good correlation between high levels of TNF and the outcome of falciparum malaria. TNF production and release could account for the fever, leukocytosis, enhanced sequestration, hypoglycaemia, dyserythropoeisis and possibly even the impaired consciousness observed in malaria. Other cytokines such as many of the interleukins and γ-interferon may also have a role to play which may sometimes be synergistic (Table 2: see Chapter 9: The biology of malarial fever). Another mediator released in response to TNF is phospholipase A2 (PLA2), a molecule central to many of the consequences of the 'sepsis syndrome' and presumably to the inflammation of malaria (Vadas et al, 1993).

Table 2. Changes in cytokines and their receptors in malaria.

Cytokine	Change	Reference
IL-1, TNF, IFN-γ	Increased	Kwiatkowski et al (1989)
TNF receptor	Increased	Kern et al (1992)
IL-2, cell bound IL-2R	Not increased	Ho et al (1988)
Soluble IL-2	Increased	Jakobsen et al (1994)
IL-3	Not increased	Ringwald et al (1993)
IL-6	Increased	Kern et al (1989)
IL-8	Increased	Friedland et al (1993)
IL-10	Increased	Peyron et al (1994)
Soluble ELAM	Increased	Wenisch et al (1994b)
ICAM, TNF receptor		
Soluble VCAM	Increased	Wenisch et al (1994a)
GM-CSF	Not increased	Ringwald et al (1993)

Abbreviations: IFN-γ interferon-γ; ELAM, endothelial leukocyte adhesion molecule; GM-CSF, granulocyte macrophage colony stimulating factor.

The use of falciparum malaria earlier this century in the treatment of syphilis would indicate that disease severity is related to the 'strain' of parasite employed. In vitro at least, different parasite lines vary in their capacity to stimulate TNF from macrophages (Allan et al, 1993). It is not known whether this observation is due to a quantitative or qualitative attribute of the toxin or how the toxin of other species of malaria, sometimes leading to comparable TNF levels, results in relatively benign disease.

FACTORS IN THE HOST

Innate

Human populations living in areas endemic for malaria have been exposed to the selective pressure of fatal malaria for many generations. Thus, malarial disease occurs on the background of a vast range of genetic polymorphisms involving the red cell and components of the human immune system which may modify outcome. The acute phase response may well provide such protection, and one study at least has shown that α-1 acidglycoprotein (AGP), inhibits the invasion of P. falciparum into red cells (Friedman, 1983).

Red cell variants

Many red cell variants affecting the membrane (Melanesian ovalocytosis), haemoglobin (haemoglobinopathies, e.g. Hb S, C, E etc.) or red cell enzymes (e.g. glucose-6 phosphate dehydrogenase (G6PD) deficiency) are argued to provide relative protection against severe malarial disease and death (Nagel, 1990). The mechanisms by which these variants might protect also vary, e.g. decreased invasion of ovalocytic cells (Kidson et al, 1981), retarded parasite growth in cells containing Hb F and Hb S (Pasvol et al, 1978), increased binding of immunoglobulin to the surface of infected cells in the case of thalassaemia (Luzzi et al, 1991), and oxidant sensitivity in the case of G6PD-deficiency.

Class I and II major histocompatibility loci

A case control study in The Gambia in West Africa has suggested an association between protection against both cerebral malaria and malarial anaemia and the presence of the HLA class I antigen HLA-B53, and protection against malarial anaemia by a class II haplotype (DRB1*1302-DQB1*0501: Hill et al, 1991, 1992). However, the same associations have not been found in East Africa for class I or II antigens where a significant protective association with a different, as yet unpublished, HLA-DR type has been identified (Hill et al, 1994).

Tumour necrosis factor

Whilst the red cell and MHC variants described above are thought to be associated with clinical protection, a recent study has ascribed susceptibility to cerebral malaria to the TNF2 allele, a variant of the TNF-α gene promoter region (McGuire et al, 1994). The TNF2 polymorphism is located at the −308 nucleotide upstream of the start of the TNF gene and has been associated with higher constitutive and inducible levels of transcription compared to the TNF1 allele. Homozygotes for the TNF2 allele were found to have a seven-fold risk of death and severe neurological sequelae from cerebral malaria when compared to those without the allele. However, it has not as yet been established that TNF2 homozygotes with malaria do indeed exhibit elevated TNF levels.

Acquired

Many acquired host factors relate to the outcome of malaria. Only a few are briefly enumerated.

Immunity

Acquisition of immunity to malaria undoubtedly has a profound effect on the clinical outcome of infection. The facts that immunity is broadly strain-specific and that falciparum parasites are antigenically highly diverse, have served to explain the prolonged period of exposure that appears to be required for the expression of protective immunity in endemic populations. This view has recently been challenged by studies in Indonesia where, contrary to common belief, the age of the individual appears to be relatively more important than the duration of exposure in the acquisition of protective immunity (Baird et al, 1993).

The mechanisms by which immunity is acquired, maintained and acts to reduce infection and disease remain largely unknown. A few deserve mention. Low grade persistent infections appear to maintain immunity (premunition). Changes in the parasite population in the infected individual would seem to correlate with disease. The study of these changes which is now feasible through the use of PCR (Viriyakosol et al, 1994), might help explain how protective immunity is acquired. The importance of antibody-mediated uptake of infected cells by the reticuloendothelial system as a major protective mechanism also needs to be corroborated. The absence of fulminating falciparum malaria in HIV infection also needs to be explored in greater detail in order to shed light on the role of T cells in the acquisition of immunity.

Age

Whilst in endemic areas it is young children who are mostly at risk of severe disease and death, in non-immune cases exposed for the first time as adults, it would appear that the risk of death increases with age especially in the elderly (Sabatinelli et al, 1994), and in the presence of underlying conditions, e.g. ischaemic heart disease, chronic lung disease and diabetes.

Pregnancy

The risk of developing severe malaria and dying is increased in pregnancy; most dramatically in primiparae and is presumably due to immunosuppression (Brabin and Brabin, 1992).

Superinfection

Patients with malaria are immunosuppressed and, in addition to their malaria may have further complicating infections due to gram positive (e.g. *Streptococcus pneumoniae*), or Gram-negative (e.g. *E. coli* and *Salmonellae* spp.) organisms. Secondary bacterial infections may account for the so called 'algid' malaria in which patients with malaria present with hypotension and shock.

Mixed malarial infection

In endemic areas the population is frequently exposed to infection by more than a single malaria parasite species. Studies on the prevalence of mixed infection using PCR, which can detect even a single parasite in a sample, have demonstrated an unexpectedly high frequency with which mixed infections occur (Snounou et al, 1993). In a preliminary study, children with *P. falciparum* alone were more likely to be febrile than children with mixed *P. falciparum* and *P. malariae* infection (Black et al, 1994). This observation may indicate that, contrary to current belief, cross-protection between parasite species, leading to less severe disease, may occur.

Nutrition

Nutritional status, iron deficiency and their relationship to severe malaria remain uncertain despite many studies on the subject (Greenwood et al, 1991).

ENVIRONMENTAL 'HUMAN' FACTORS

It may well be asked why deaths should still occur in a disease which can be relatively easily diagnosed and for which adequate, although not perfect, anti-malarial drugs exist. Unfortunately, even with the best intentions and under relatively good conditions, deaths from malaria due to human error remain a reality.

Delay in treatment

One of the main associations with disease severity and mortality appears to be delay in treatment, especially where the illness is not recognized as malaria and is mistaken for another such as influenza, infectious diarrhoea, a respiratory tract infection or hepatitis. However, there are still a number of patients in whom the onset is abrupt, convulsions and coma set in rapidly and these people are at the greatest risk of death in the first few hours after admission to hospital regardless of what intervention is undertaken. In this respect malaria may be analagous to meningitis; there are those patients in whom the onset is insidious and the course is relatively mild, those in whom the onset is acute but non-fulminant and where prompt treatment is critical, and those with a fulminant course, who die early regardless of any intervention (Radetsky, 1992).

Failure of prophylaxis

Delay in treatment often results when the likelihood of malaria is not considered in the face of either erratic or even compliant anti-malarial prophylaxis. No anti-malarial regimen provides total protection, and where there is drug resistance severe disease can evolve even when on full prophylaxis, although breakthrough disease on prophylaxis tends to be milder (Lewis et al, 1992).

Iatrogenic

In a small number of cases, patients with severe malaria die not of the disease but because of treatment. Iatrogenic cause of death remains a reality, largely unconfessed and often unknowing. The main drugs used, i.e. chloroquine and quinine, both have potentially lethal side effects. Chloroquine when injected rapidly and at a high dose intravenously can lead to dramatic hypotension and arrhythmias, as can quinine (Winstanley, 1992). Quinine has the added problem of being a potent stimulant of insulin secretion leading to severe hypoglycaemia and, in a few cases, has led to fatal tetanus when given intramuscularly (Yen et al, 1994). Rapid over-hydration in the erroneous belief that patients with malaria are dehydrated, in whom pulmonary capillary damage may exist and who are more often that not hypoalbuminaemic, can lead to pulmonary oedema. The former practice of high dose steroid infusion for severe malaria has led to fatality due to massive gastroenterological bleeding or superinfection in a small number of cases (Warrell et al, 1982).

OVERALL PATHOGENIC MECHANISMS

It would be naive to contemplate that the above-mentioned factors of host, parasite or environment act in isolation. A model of malarial pathogenesis would need to take into account the delicate interplay between many of these factors (see Table 1). In any event the relationships might be far more complex. For example, in the debate of whether the cerebral manifestations of falciparum malaria are due to the obstruction of small vessels by sequestered parasites leading to reduced perfusion and hypoxia, or due to toxin-induced release of mediators, both mechanisms might be equally relevant. Sequestration would not only lead to microvascular obstruction but could also serve to localize the effect of these mediators. The factors determining which particular complications of malarial disease will predominate often do not follow intuition. However, in a discussion of pathogenesis, three important clinical entities merit separate mention, namely cerebral malaria, anaemia and respiratory distress.

Cerebral malaria

In cerebral malaria there appears to be no reduction in total cerebral blood flow, although blood flow is low relative to the cerebral arterial oxygen content (Warrell et al, 1988). Cerebral malaria can occur in the absence of a localized inflammatory cell response, direct tissue invasion (MacPherson et al, 1985), a breakdown in the blood–brain barrier (Warrell et al, 1986), cerebral oedema (Newton et al, 1994), disseminated intravascular coagulation, hypoglycaemia or any microscopic evidence of an immunopathological mechanism for the observed cerebral dysfunction (MacPherson et al, 1985). None of the cerebrospinal fluid parameters such as a pleocytosis or increased protein as is found in meningitis or encephalitis, occur in cerebral malaria, except for a raised lactate. At post mortem, apart from pigmentation due to haemozoin resulting from the breakdown of haemoglobin, the occasional petechial haemorrhage and other minor findings, the brain appears to be relatively normal with little extravascular pathology (MacPherson et al, 1985). There is no inflammatory cell infiltrate, the vascular system is generally intact and, despite the popular concept of cerebral malaria being the result of small vessel occlusion by parasitized cells, macro- or microinfarction of tissue is not a major feature of patients dying with the disease. Moreover the majority of patients who recover from unrousable coma due to malaria appear to suffer few, if any, neurological sequelae, quite unlike any other neurological infection in man of equal severity.

There is remarkably little extravascular pathology in patients who die of malaria. Small microhaemorrhages may occur around capillaries and venules but there are few platelets or microthrombi evident. Instead, the syndrome appears to be related to the tight packing of schizonts in the small capillaries of the brain, a process brought about by sequestration, which in turn results from one or a combination of cytoadherence, rosetting or the decreased deformability of infected cells (Cranston et al, 1984).

More recently the occurrence of raised intracranial pressure has been invoked in the pathogenesis of cerebral malaria in children (Newton et al, 1991). In East Africa the CSF opening pressure was raised in the 26 children studied who had cerebral malaria, and all children who died showed clinical evidence of a central or uncal herniation syndrome in which the brain stem appeared to be progressively compressed through the tentorial notch. None of those children who manifested evidence of lower brain stem compression recovered. Doppler studies of the middle cerebral artery showed reversal of blood flow in diastole, characteristic of a central herniation syndrome. Clark et al (1992) have hypothesized that the local release of nitric oxide (NO) by endothelial cells in the brain leads to inhibition of neurotransmission and coma. NO, by causing vasodilatation, may also increase intracranial pressure by increasing intracranial blood volume. However, the role of NO is at present only a hypothetical one (Kremsner et al, 1993).

Anaemia

The pathophysiology of the anaemia of falciparum malaria is both complex and multifactorial (Abdalla et al, 1980; Phillips and Pasvol, 1992), and results in a condition which is a major cause of mortality and morbidity in patients, especially children and pregnant women. The importance of anaemia as a cause of death in malaria may well be underestimated because of difficulty in diagnosis, especially where parasitaemia may be low and the clinical picture may be confused with other causes of anaemia.

In the anaemia due to malaria the fall in haemoglobin is often far in excess of what can be accounted for by the loss of infected red blood cells alone. Two clinical presentations predominate; severe acute malaria in which anaemia supervenes (Phillips et al, 1986), and severe anaemia in patients in whom the illness has developed insidiously (Abdalla et al, 1980). In the first, patients suffering a severe acute attack of malaria and who are seen early after the onset of the clinical symptoms, are initially not anaemic, nor do they have splenomegaly. However, anaemia develops, often dramatically, during the subsequent course of the infection. The causes of anaemia in malaria in these acute episodes are multifactorial and might differ according to the stage of the malaria infection. In a study of uncomplicated falciparum malaria, patients seen within 24 to 48 hours of the onset of fever were usually not anaemic, but there was a steady fall in haematocrit over the next 4 or 5 days which continued well after the peripheral blood parasitaemia had been cleared (Phillips et al, 1986). Uninfected red cells were of normal shape, size and colour without evidence of fragmentation or spherocytosis. The reticulocyte response to this rapidly developing anaemia was usually brisk, but only well after the parasites had been cleared. If the parasite clearance was delayed, the reticulocyte count did not rise despite a severe progressive fall in haematocrit. This delay in reticulocyte response associated with persistent parasitaemia would suggest that the parasites themselves are in some way responsible for the sustained inhibition of erythropoiesis or for suppression of the release of erythroid cells into the peripheral circulation, perhaps via TNF-dependent mechanisms (Clark and Chaudhri, 1988). This observation fits in well with the sustained bone marrow suppression that is observed in the context of trypanosomiasis in mice, and which is believed to be the result of NO-induced suppression of erythroid precursors (Mabbott and Sternberg, 1995).

Three phases in which the haematocrit falls during treatment of acute malaria have been identified (Phillips et al, 1986). The first is as a result of rehydration, the second correlates with the fall in parasitaemia and the third indicates a loss of uninfected cells. The marked persistence of anaemia in this acute setting has been related to a combination of shortened survival of uninfected cells (Looareesuwan et al, 1987) and evidence of bone marrow suppression (Srichaikul et al, 1967, 1969; Srichaikul and Siriasawakul, 1976).

The second pattern of development of anaemia in the context of malaria occurs in endemic areas in particular (Abdalla et al, 1980). These patients, usually children, are clearly anaemic when first seen. The history is usually one of intermittent fevers and general symptoms of ill health occurring insidiously over weeks rather than days. Splenomegaly of varying degree is present and the peripheral blood film shows scanty asexual parasitaemia.

The bone marrow often shows the picture of dyserythropoiesis (Abdalla et al, 1980), a morphological appearance, which in functional terms results in ineffective erythropoiesis. In many cases gametocytaemia and malarial pigment in phagocytic cells are seen, evidence of a past rather than current attack of malaria. Attributing the cause of anaemia in this setting is often difficult, and some sources have included a minimal arbitrary haemoglobin level and parasitaemia count (< 5 gm/dl in the presence of parasitaemia of more than $10\,000/\mu$l) to define malarial anaemia. This definition should however, be regarded as being for research rather than clinical purposes.

Sequential studies have emphasized the difficulty of analysing the various mechanisms that contribute to the development of the anaemia of malaria. There is still no comprehensive understanding of the relative contributions made by intravascular haemolysis, extravascular clearance of red blood cells and marrow dysfunction, but a clearer picture is beginning to emerge. The major mechanisms are those of red cell destruction and decreased red cell production. The former include loss of infected cells by rupture or phagocytosis, removal of uninfected cells due to antibody sensitization or other physicochemical membrane changes and increased reticuloendothelial activity, particularly in organs such as the spleen and bone marrow (Abdalla et al, 1980; Phillips and Pasvol, 1992). Shortened red cell survival may persist well after parasite clearance (Looareesuwan et al, 1987). Decreased production results from marrow hypoplasia seen in acute infections (Srichaikul et al, 1967, 1969; Srichaikul and Siriasawakul, 1976), and dyserythropoiesis seen in more prolonged infections (Abdalla et al, 1980). The role of parvovirus as a possible cause of bone marrow aplasia in a few cases has been postulated (Jones et al, 1990). It has recently been suggested that antibodies to a glycolytic pathway enzyme, triosephosphate isomerase (TPI) may be involved, but how these antibodies act is difficult in view of TPI being an intracellular molecule (Ritter et al, 1993). The raised activity of PLA2 observed in malaria has also been implicated in haemolysis as this enzyme can lyse infected red cells (Vadas et al, 1993).

Respiratory distress

To anyone who has cared for patients with severe malaria in an endemic area, or in the non-immune after travel abroad, the observation of respiratory distress of one kind or another is not infrequent. Respiratory distress and abnormal rhythms of respiration are common in African children who die of malaria (Marsh et al, 1995), and we have observed tachypnoea and hiccoughs in patients with imported severe malaria. It remains unclear whether these manifestations are due to pulmonary/diaphragmatic or cerebral irritation. Respiratory distress may be defined at two levels; the first, a particularly loose one, is the response of a clinician to the question 'Does the patient have respiratory distress?' The second, more restrictive definition, includes only those patients (largely children) with documented intercostal recession or acidotic breathing. As with so many complications of malaria, the cause of this respiratory distress, which may well contribute to mortality, appears to be multifold and remains poorly understood. First, it may be the respiratory component of a mechanism to compensate for the metabolic acidosis which can accompany severe disease (Taylor et al, 1993). Second, it may be due to the direct effects of the parasite or raised intracranial pressure on the respiratory centre in the brain stem. Third, there may be secondary lung infection as a consequence of immunosuppression. Fourth, there may be air hunger as a result of severe anaemia. Finally there may be pulmonary oedema as a consequence of hypoalbuminaemia, iatrogenic fluid overload, direct alveolar capillary damage by parasites and neutrophils leading to the acute respiratory distress syndrome. The ultrastructure in the lung of patients with malaria shows that the main pathological finding is that of neutrophils and the presence of rings or trophozoites rather than schizonts (Duarte et al, 1985; MacPherson et al, 1985)

Other manifestations

Many of the other complications of malaria are described in Chapter 4: The clinical manifestations and diagnosis of malaria. The occurrence of hypoglycaemia is an important complication of malaria and is of multifactorial causation; depletion of stores largely because of starvation and/or malnutrition, malabsorption of glucose because of decreased splanchnic blood flow, increased tissue metabolism, parasite utilization of glucose, impaired gluconeogenesis and hyperinsulinaemia due to quinine therapy. The metabolism of glucose results in the production of lactate leading to severe acidaemia. Acidaemia (blood pH less than 7.3) and lactic acidosis have recently been shown to be two of the most important prognostic factors in severe malaria (Taylor et al 1993; Krishna et al, 1994). Acidaemia has been shown to be associated with respiratory rhythm abnormalities (especially a slow respiratory rhythm) and death. Other important complications of severe malaria include blackwater fever, renal failure and disseminated intravascular coagulation, as well as more subtle activation of the coagulation cascade with a reduction in antithrombin III, elevation in thrombin–antithrombin III complexes and reduction in factor XII and prekallikrein activities (Clemens et al, 1994). The mechanisms leading to many of these complications are the least well documented and remain an important area for future research.

SUMMARY

Over a quarter of the world's population remains at risk of malaria and up to 250 million clinical cases occur each year of which over 1 million will die of *Plasmodium falciparum* infection. Why so many individuals are infected, but only relatively few proceed to severe disease such as cerebral malaria, severe anaemia or respiratory distress, remains poorly understood.

A number of parasite–host interactions are important in the pathogenesis of severe falciparum malaria. One of the major determinants of parasite density, often related to disease severity, is the ability of the merozoite to invade red cells. The red cell glycophorins and at least one parasite component, EBA 175, appear to be involved. Adherence of parasitized red cells to endothelium (cytoadherence) is a feature of falciparum malaria and may serve to concentrate the effects of the parasite locally. The binding of uninfected red cells to parasitized red cells (rosetting) is one parasite phenotype that shows an association with disease severity. Whilst rosetting may increase sequestration of the parasitized cell in small vessels, it does not appear to enhance invasion. The production of a toxin (or toxins) by the parasite is currently favoured as a major pathogenic mechanism, but the conclusive identity and characterization of such molecules have yet to be resolved.

Falciparum malaria in man occurs against the background of many genetic polymorphisms involving the red cell variants, the MHC complex, the TNF promoter and doubtless many others as yet undiscovered. Acquired factors such as the state of immunity of the individual, age, pregnancy, superinfection, mixed malarial infections and nutrition may influence disease severity and outcome. However, in a consideration of why patients with falciparum malaria continue to die, human factors which include a delay in seeking treatment, failure of prophylaxis and iatrogenically induced disease, cannot be omitted.

In the pathogenesis of severe disease a number of anomalies exist. In cerebral malaria there is no consistent reduction in total cerebral blood flow, no marked inflammatory cell response, no tissue invasion or necrosis, no breakdown in the blood–brain barrier, no cerebral oedema, no disseminated intravascular coagulation or hypoglycaemia. Instead schizont-infected cells are packed or sequestered into the capillaries of the brain as a result of cytoadherence, rosetting and changes in red cell deformability. Raised intracranial pressure may also play a role leading to herniation of the brain stem and death. The role of NO in the coma of cerebral malaria remains an attractive hypothesis. Malarial anaemia, whilst primarily a result of haemolysis, also encompasses impaired red cell production. Respiratory distress, a newly identified feature of severe disease, will almost certainly prove to have a number of underlying causes and be of importance in assessing prognosis.

Acknowledgements

We would like to thank Drs RN Davidson and RJ Wilkinson for their critical comments. BC is supported by the Wellcome Trust.

REFERENCES

Abdalla S, Weatherall D, Wickramasinghe S & Hughes M (1980) The anaemia of *P. falciparum* malaria. *British Journal of Haematology* **46:** 171–183.

Allan RJ, Rowe A & Kwiatkowski D (1993) *Plasmodium falciparum* varies in its ability to induce tumor necrosis factor. *Infection and Immunity* **61:** 4772–4776.

Baird JK, Purnomo, Basri H et al (1993) Age-specific prevalence of *Plasmodium falciparum* among six populations with limited histories of exposure to endemic malaria. *American Journal of Tropical Medicine and Hygiene* **49:** 707–719.

Bate C & Kwiatkowski D (1994) Stimulators of tumour necrosis factor production released by damaged erythrocytes. *Immunology* **83:** 256–261.

Bate CA, Taverne J, Roman E et al (1992) Tumour necrosis factor induction by malaria exoantigens depends upon phospholipid. *Immunology* **75:** 129–135.

Berendt AR, Simmons DL, Tansey J et al (1989) Intercellular adhesion molecule-1 is an endothelial cell adhesion receptor for *Plasmodium falciparum*. *Nature* **341:** 57–59.

Berendt A, Ferguson D & Newbold C (1990) Sequestration in *Plasmodium falciparum* malaria: sticky cells and sticky problems. *Parasitology Today* **6:** 247–254.

Black J, Hommel M, Snounou G & Pinder M (1994) Mixed infections with *Plasmodium falciparum* and *P. malariae* and fever in malaria. *Lancet* **343:** 1095.

Bouharoun TH, Attanath P, Sabchareon A et al (1990) Antibodies that protect humans against *Plasmodium falciparum* blood stages do not on their own inhibit parasite growth and invasion in vitro, but act in cooperation with monocytes. *Journal of Experimental Medicine* **172:** 1633–1641.

Brabin L & Brabin B (1992) Parasitic infections in women and their consequences. *Advances in Parasitology* **31:** 1–81.

Carlson J & Wahlgren M (1992) *Plasmodium falciparum* erythrocyte rosetting is mediated by promiscuous lectin-like interactions. *Journal of Experimental Medicine* **176:** 1311–1317.

Carlson J, Helmby H, Hill AVS et al (1990a) Human cerebral malaria: association with erythrocyte rosetting and lack of anti-rosetting antibodies. *Lancet* **336:** 1457–1460.

Carlson J, Holmquist G, Taylor DW et al (1990b) Antibodies to a histidine-rich protein (PfHRP1) disrupt spontaneously formed *Plasmodium falciparum* erythrocyte rosettes. *Proceedings of the National Academy of Sciences of the USA* **87:** 2511–2515.

Clark I & Chaudhri G (1988) Tumour necrosis factor may contribute to the anaemia of malaria by causing dyserythropoiesis and erythrophagocytosis. *British Journal of Haematology* **70:** 99–103.

Clark IA, Chaudhri G & Cowden WB (1989) Roles of tumour necrosis factor in the illness and pathology of malaria. *Transactions of the Royal Society of Tropical Medicine and Hygiene* **83:** 436–440.

Clark IA, Rockett KA & Cowden WB (1992) Possible central role of nitric oxide in conditions clinically similar to cerebral malaria. *Lancet* **340:** 894–896.

Clemens R, Pramoolsinsap C, Lorenz R et al (1994) Activation of the coagulation cascade in severe falciparum malaria through the intrinsic pathway. *British Journal of Haematology* **87:** 100–105.

Clough B, Paulitschke M, Nash G et al (1995) Mechanism of regulation of malarial invasion by extraerythrocytic ligands. *Molecular and Biochemical Parasitology* **69:** 19–27.

Cooke B, Berendt A, Craig A et al (1994) Rolling and stationary cytoadhesion of red blood cells parasitized by *Plasmodium falciparum*: separate roles for ICAM-1, CD36 and thrombospondin. *British Journal of Haematology* **87:** 162–170.

Cranston HA, Boylan CW, Carroll GL et al (1984) *Plasmodium falciparum* maturation abolishes physiologic red cell deformability. *Science* **223:** 400–403.

David P, Handunetti S, Leech J et al (1988) Uninfected erythrocytes form 'rosettes' around *Plasmodium falciparum* infected erythrocytes. *American Journal of Tropical Medicine and Hygiene* **38:** 289–297.

Dolan SA, Miller LH & Wellems TE (1990) Evidence for a switching mechanism in the invasion of erythrocytes by *Plasmodium falciparum*. *Journal of Clinical Investigation* **86:** 618–624.

Duarte MI, Corbett CE, Boulos M & Amato NV (1985) Ultrastructure of the lung in falciparum malaria. *American Journal of Tropical Medicine and Hygiene* **34:** 31–35.

Erunkulu E, Hill A, Kwiatkowski D et al (1992) Severe malaria in Gambian children is not due to lack of previous exposure to malaria. *Clinical and Experimental Immunlogy* **89:** 296–300.

Esslinger CW, Picot S & Ambroise TP (1994) Intra-erythrocytic *Plasmodium falciparum* induces up-regulation of inter-cellular adhesion molecule-1 on human endothelial cells in vitro. *Scandanavian Journal of Immunology* **39:** 229–232.

Friedland JS, Ho M, Remick DG et al (1993) Interleukin-8 and *Plasmodium falciparum* malaria in Thailand. *Transactions of the Royal Society of Hygiene and Tropical Medicine* **87:** 54–55.

Friedman MJ (1983) Control of malaria virulence by alpha 1-acid glycoprotein (orosomucoid), an acute-phase (inflammatory) reactant. *Proceedings of the National Academy of Sciences of the USA* **80:** 5421–5424.

Gerold P, Dieckmann-Schuppert A & Schwarz RT (1994) Glycosylphosphatidylinositols synthesized by asexual erythrocytic stages of the malarial parasite, *Plasmodium falciparum*. Candidates for plasmodial glycosylphosphatidylinositol membrane anchor precursors and pathogenicity factors. *Journal of Biological Chemistry* **269**: 2597–2606.

Goldring JD, Molyneux ME, Taylor T et al (1992) *Plasmodium falciparum*: diversity of isolates from Malawi in their cytoadherence to melanoma cells and monocytes in vitro. *British Journal of Haematology* **81**: 413–418.

Grau G & de Kossodo S (1994) Role of cytokines and adhesion molecules in malaria: protection versus pathology. In Griffin G (ed.) *Baillière's Clinical Infectious Diseases*, pp 75–95. London: Baillière Tindall.

Greenwood B, Marsh K & Snow R (1991) Why do some African children develop severe malaria? *Parasitology Today* **7**: 277–281.

Hadley TA, Klotz FW, Pasvol G et al (1987) Falciparum malaria parasites invade erythrocytes that lack glycophorin A and B (MkMk). *The Journal of Clinical Investigation* **80**: 1190–1193.

Handunnetti SM, David PH, Perera KLRL & Mendis KN (1989) Uninfected erythrocytes form 'Rosettes' around *Plasmodium falciparum* infected erythrocytes. *American Journal of Tropical Medicine and Hygiene* **40**: 115–118.

Handunnetti SM, van SM, Hasler T et al (1992) Involvement of CD36 on erythrocytes as a rosetting receptor for *Plasmodium falciparum*-infected erythrocytes. *Blood* **80**: 2097–2104.

Harpaz R, Edelman R, Wasserman SS et al (1992) Serum cytokine profiles in experimental human malaria. Relationship to protection and disease course after challenge. *The Journal of Clinical Investigation* **90**: 515–523.

Hasler T, Handunnetti SM, Aguiar JC et al (1990) In vitro rosetting, cytoadherence, and micro-agglutination properties of *Plasmodium falciparum*-infected erythrocytes from Gambian and Tanzanian patients. *Blood* **76**: 1845–1852.

Helmby H, Cavelier L, Pettersson U & Wahlgren M (1993) Rosetting *Plasmodium falciparum*-infected erythrocytes express unique strain-specific antigens on their surface. *Infection and Immunity* **61**: 284–288.

Hill A, Allsopp C, Kwiatkowski D et al (1991) Common West African HLA antigens are associated with protection from severe malaria. *Nature* **352**: 595–600.

Hill A, Yates S, Allsopp C et al (1994) Human leukocyte antigens and natural selection by malaria. *Philosophical Transactions of the Royal Society of London B* **346**: 379–385.

Hill AV, Elvin J, Willis AC et al (1992) Molecular analysis of the association of HLA-B53 and resistance to severe malaria. *Nature* **360**: 434–439.

Ho M, Webster H, Looareesuwan S et al (1988) Defective production of and response to interleukin 2 in acute falciparum malaria. *Journal of Immunology* **141**: 2755–2759.

Ho M, Davis TME, Silamut K et al (1991) Rosette formation of *Plasmodium falciparum*-infected erythrocytes from patients with acute malaria. *Infection and Immunity* **59**: 2135–2139.

Jakobsen PH, Morris JS, Theander TG et al (1994) Increased plasma levels of soluble IL-2R are associated with severe *Plasmodium falciparum* malaria. *Clinical and Experimental Immunology* **96**: 98–103.

Jones P, Pickett L, Anderson M & Pasvol G (1990) Human parvovirus infection in children and severe anaemia seen in an area endemic for malaria. *Journal of Tropical Medicine and Hygiene* **93**: 67–70.

Kain KC, Orlandi PA, Haynes JD et al (1993) Evidence for two-stage binding by the 175-kD erythrocyte binding antigen of *Plasmodium falciparum*. *Journal of Experimental Medicine* **178**: 1497–1505.

Kaul D, Roth E, Nagel R et al (1991) Rosetting of *Plasmodium falciparum* infected red blood cells with uninfected red blood cells enhances microvascular obstruction under flow conditions. *Blood* **78**: 812–819.

Kern P, Hemmer CJ, Van DJ et al (1989) Elevated tumor necrosis factor alpha and interleukin-6 serum levels as markers for complicated *Plasmodium falciparum* malaria. *American Journal of Medicine* **87**: 139–143.

Kern P, Hemmer CJ, Gallati H et al (1992) Soluble tumor necrosis factor receptors correlate with parasitemia and disease severity in human malaria. *Journal of Infectious Diseases* **166**: 930–934.

Kidson C, Lamont G, Saul A & Nurse GT (1981) Ovalocytic erythrocytes from Melanesians are resistant to invasion by malaria parasites in culture. *Proceedings of the National Academy of Sciences of the USA* **78**: 5829–5832.

Kremsner PG, Nussler A, Neifer S et al (1993) Malaria antigen and cytokine-induced production of reactive nitrogen intermediates by murine macrophages: no relevance to the development of experimental cerebral malaria. *Immunology* **78**: 286–290.

Krishna S, Waller DW, ter Kuile F et al (1994) Lactic acidosis and hypoglycaemia in children with severe malaria: pathophysiological and prognostic significance. *Transactions of the Royal Society of Tropical Medicine and Hygiene* **88:** 67–73.

Kwiatkowski D, Cannon JG, Manogue KR et al (1989) Tumour necrosis factor production in falciparum malaria and its association with schizont rupture. *Clinical and Experimental Parasitology* **77:** 361–366.

Lewis SJ, Davidson RN, Ross EJ & Hall AP (1992) Severity of imported falciparum malaria: effect of taking antimalarial prophylaxis. *British Medical Journal* **305:** 741–743.

Looareesuwan S, Merry A, Phillips R et al (1987) Reduced erythrocyte survival following clearance of malarial parasitaemia in Thai patients. *British Journal of Haematology* **67:** 473–478.

Luzzi GA, Merry AH, Newbold CI et al (1991) Surface antigen expression on *Plasmodium falciparum*-infected erythrocytes is modified in alpha- and beta-thalassemia. *Journal of Experimental Medicine* **173:** 785–791.

Mabbott N & Sternberg J (1995) Bone marrow nitric oxide production and the development of anemia in *Trypanosoma brucei*-infected mice *Infection and Immunity* **63:** 1563–1566.

MacPherson G, Warrell M, White N et al (1985) Human cerebral malaria. A quantitative ultrastructural analysis of parasitised erythrocyte sequestration. *American Journal of Pathology* **119:** 385–401.

Marsh K, Marsh VM, Brown J et al (1988) *Plasmodium falciparum*: the behavior of clinical isolates in an in vitro model of infected red blood cell sequestration. *Experimental Parasitology* **65:** 202–208.

Marsh K, Forster D, Waruira C et al (1995) Indicators of life-threatening malaria in African children. *New England Journal of Medicine* **332:** 1399–1404.

McElroy P, Beier J, Oster C et al (1994) Predicting outcome in malaria: correlation between rate of exposure to infected mosquitoes and level of *Plasmodium falciparum* parasitemia. *American Journal of Tropical Medicine and Hygiene* **51:** 523–532.

McGuire W, Hill A, Allsopp C et al (1994) Variation in the TNF-α promoter region associated with susceptibility to cerebral malaria. *Nature* **371:** 508–511.

Nagel RL (1990) Innate resistance to malaria: the intraerythrocytic cycle. *Blood Cells* **16:** 321–339.

Newton CR, Kirkham FJ, Winstanley PA et al (1991) Intracranial pressure in African children with cerebral malaria. *Lancet* **337:** 573–576.

Newton CR, Peshu N, Kendall B et al (1994) Brain swelling and ischaemia in Kenyans with cerebral malaria. *Archives of the Diseases of Childhood* **70:** 281–287.

Ockenhouse CF, Tegoshi T, Maeno Y et al (1992) Human vascular endothelial cell adhesion receptors for *Plasmodium falciparum*-infected erythrocytes: roles for endothelial leukocyte adhesion molecule 1 and vascular cell adhesion molecule 1. *Journal of Experimental Medicine* **176:** 1183–1189.

Orlandi PA, Klotz FW & Haynes JD (1992) A malaria invasion receptor, the 175-kilodalton erythrocyte binding antigen of *Plasmodium falciparum* recognizes the terminal Neu5Ac(α2-3)Gal-sequences of glycophorin A. *The Journal of Cell Biology* **116:** 901–909.

Pasvol G (1984) Receptors on red cells for *Plasmodium falciparum* and their interaction with merozoites. *Philosophical Transactions of the Royal Society of London* **307:** 189–200.

Pasvol G, Weatherall DJ & Wilson RJ (1978) Cellular mechanism for the protective effect of haemoglobin S against *Plasmodium falciparum* malaria. *Nature* **274:** 701–703.

Pasvol G, Weatherall DJ & Wilson RJ (1980) The increased susceptibility of young red cells to invasion by the malarial parasite *Plasmodium falciparum*. *British Journal of Haematology* **45:** 285–295.

Pasvol G, Jungery M, Weatherall DJ et al (1982) Glycophorin as a possible receptor for *Plasmodium falciparum*. *Lancet* **ii:** 947–950.

Pasvol G, Hodson C, Tanner MJA & Newbold CI (1987) The relative roles of N- and O-linked carbohydrate in the invasion of human red cells by merozoites of *Plasmodium falciparum*. In Chang K-P & Snary D (eds) *Host–Parasite Cellular and Molecular Interactions in Protozoal Infections*, pp 245–254. Springer-Verlag: Berlin, Heidelberg.

Pasvol G, Chasis JA, Mohandas N et al (1989) Inhibition of malarial parasite invasion by monoclonal antibodies against glycophorin A correlates with reduction in red cell membrane deformability. *Blood* **74:** 1836–1843.

Pasvol G, Clough B & Carlsson J (1992) Malaria and the red cell membrane. *Blood Reviews* **6:** 183–192.

Pasvol G, Carlsson J & Clough B (1993) The red cell membrane and invasion by malarial parasites. In Tanner M & Anstee D (eds) *Baillière's Clinical Haematology*, pp 513–534. London: Baillière Tindall.

Perkins ME (1991) Approaches to study merozoite invasion of erythrocytes. *Research in Immunology* 142: 662–665.

Peyron F, Burdin N, Ringwald P et al (1994) High levels of circulating IL-10 in human malaria. *Clinical and Experimental Immunology* 95: 300–303.

Phillips R & Pasvol G (1992) Anaemia of *Plasmodium falciparum* malaria. *Baillière's Clinical Haematology* pp 315–330. London: Baillière Tindall.

Phillips R, Looareesuwan S, Warrell D et al (1986) The importance of anaemia in cerebral and uncomplicated falciparum malaria: role of complications, dyserythropoiesis and iron sequestration. *Quarterly Journal of Medicine* 58: 305–323.

Pichyangkul S, Saengkrai P & Webster H (1994) *Plasmodium falciparum* pigment induces monocytes to release high levels of tumor necrosis factor-α and interleukin-1β. *American Journal of Tropical Medicine and Hygiene* 51: 430–435.

Radetsky M (1992) Duration of symptoms and outcome in bacterial meningitis: an analysis of causation and the implications of a delay in diagnosis. *Paediatric Infectious Diseases Journal* 11: 694–698.

Ringwald P, Peyron F, Lepers JP et al (1993) Parasite virulence factors during falciparum malaria: rosetting, cytoadherence, and modulation of cytoadherence by cytokines. *Infection and Immunity* 61: 5198–5204.

Ritter K, Kuhlencord A, Thomssen R & Bommer W (1993) Prolonged haemolytic anaemia in malaria and autoantibodies against triosephosphate isomerase. *Lancet* 342: 1333–1334.

Roberts DD, Sherwood JA, Spitalnik SL et al (1985) Thrombospondin binds falciparum malaria parasitized erythrocytes and may mediate cytoadherence. *Nature* 318: 64–66.

Sabatinelli G, D'Ancona F, Majori G & Squarcione S (1994) Fatal malaria in Italian travellers. *Transactions of the Royal Society of Tropical Medicine and Hygiene* 88: 314.

Schofield L & Hackett F (1993) Signal transduction in host cells by a glycosylphosphatidylinositol toxin of malaria parasites. *Journal of Experimental Medicine* 177: 145–153.

Sim BKL, Orlandi PA, Haynes JD et al (1990) Primary structure of the 175K *Plasmodium falciparum* erythrocyte binding antigen and identification of a peptide which elicits antibodies that inhibit malaria merozoite invasion. *The Journal of Cell Biology* 111: 1877–1884.

Snounou G, Pinheiro L, Goncalves A et al (1993) The importance of sensitive detection of malaria parasites in the human and insect hosts in epidemiological studies, as shown by the analysis of field samples from Guinea Bissau. *Transactions of the Royal Society of Tropical Medicine and Hygiene* 87: 363–374.

Srichaikul T & Siriasawakul T (1976) Ferrokinetics in patients with malaria: haemoglobin synthesis and normoblasts in vitro. *Transactions of the Royal Society of Tropical Medicine and Hygiene* 70: 244–246.

Srichaikul T, Panikbutr N & Jeumtrakul P (1967) Bone marrow changes in human malaria. *Annals of Tropical Medicine and Parasitology* 8: 40–50.

Srichaikul T, Wasanasomsithi M & Poshyachinda V et al (1969) Ferrokinetic studies in erythropoiesis in malaria. *Archives of Internal Medicine* 124: 623–628.

Sturchler D (1989) How much malaria is there worldwide? *Parasitology Today* 5: 39–40.

Taylor TE, Borgstein A & Molyneux ME (1993) Acid-base status in paediatric *Plasmodium falciparum* malaria. *Quarterly Journal of Medicine* 86: 99–109.

Turner G, Morrison H, Jones M et al (1995) An immunohistochemical study of the pathology of malaria. Evidence for widespread endothelial activation and a role for intercellular adhesion molecule-1 in cerebral sequestration. *American Journal of Pathology* 145: 1057–1069.

Udeinya IJ, Schmidt JA, Aikawa M et al (1981) Falciparum malaria-infected erythrocytes specifically bind to cultured human endothelial cells. *Science* 213: 555–557.

Udomsangpetch R, Wåhlin B, Carlson J et al (1989) *Plasmodium falciparum*-infected erythrocytes form spontaneous erythrocyte rosettes. *Journal of Experimental Medicine* 169: 1835–1840.

Vadas P, Taylor TE, Chimsuku L et al (1993) Increased serum phospholipase A2 activity in Malawian children with falciparum malaria. *American Journal of Medicine and Tropical Medicine* 49: 455–459.

Viriyakosol S, Siripoon N, Zhu Z et al (1994) *Plasmodium falciparum*: selective growth of sub-populations from field samples following *in vitro* culture, as detected by the polymerase chain reaction. *Experimental Parasitology* 79: 517–525.

Ward G, Chitnis C & Miller L (1994) The invasion of erythrocytes by malarial parasites. In Russell D (eds) *Baillière's Clinical Infectious Diseases*, pp 155–190. London: Baillière Tindall.

Warrell D, Looareesuwan S, Warrell M et al (1982) Dexamethasone proves deleterious in cerebral malaria. A double-blind trial in 100 comatose patients. *New England Journal of Medicine* **306:** 313–319.

Warrell DA, Looareesuwan S, Phillips RE et al (1986) Function of the blood-cerebrospinal fluid barrier in human cerebral malaria: rejection of the permeability hypothesis. *American Journal of Tropical Medicine and Hygiene* **35:** 882–889.

Warrell DA, White NJ, Veall N et al (1988) Cerebral anaerobic glycolysis and reduced cerebral oxygen transport in human cerebral malaria. *Lancet* **ii:** 534–538 [Published erratum appears in *Lancet* 1988 Sept 17;2(8612):698].

Warrell D, Molyneux M & Beales P (1990) Severe and complicated malaria. *Transactions of the Royal Society of Tropical Medicine and Hygiene* **84 (supplement 2):** 1–65.

Wenisch C, Looareesuwan S, Parschalk B & Graninger W (1994a) Soluble vascular cell adhesion molecule 1 is elevated in patients with *Plasmodium falciparum* malaria. *Journal of Infectious Diseases* **169:** 710–711.

Wenisch C, Varijanonta S, Looareesuwan S et al (1994b) Soluble intercellular adhesion molecule-1 (ICAM-1), endothelial leukocyte adhesion molecule-1 (ELAM-1), and tumor necrosis factor receptor (55 kDa TNF-R) in patients with acute *Plasmodium falciparum* malaria. *Clinical Immunology and Immunopathology* **71:** 344–348.

White N (1992) The pathophysiology of malaria. *Advances in Parasitology* **31:** 83–173.

White NJ, Chapman D & Watt G (1992) The effects of multiplication and synchronicity on the vascular distribution of parasites in falciparum malaria. *Transactions of the Royal Society of Tropical Medicine and Hygiene* **86:** 590–597.

Wick TM & Louis V (1991) Cytoadherence of *Plasmodium falciparum*-infected erythrocytes to human umbilical vein and human dermal microvascular endothelial cells under shear conditions. *American Journal of Tropical Medicine and Hygiene* **45:** 578–586.

Winograd E & Sherman IW (1989) Characterization of a modified red cell membrane protein expressed on erythrocytes infected with the human malaria parasite *Plasmodium falciparum*: possible role as a cytoadherent mediating protein. *The Journal of Cell Biology* **108:** 23–30.

Winstanley PA (1992) Treatment and prevention of falciparum malaria in Africa. *Journal of the Royal College of Physicians, London* **26:** 445–449.

Yen L, Dao L, Day N et al (1994) Role of quinine in the high mortality of intramuscular injection tetanus. *Lancet* **344:** 786–787.

4

The clinical manifestations and diagnosis of malaria

MALCOLM E. MOLYNEUX

Some malarial infections are symptomless, others are fatal. Between these two extremes, malarial illness may take a variety of clinical forms differing in pattern and severity. Why plasmodia should cause such a spectrum of disease is only partially understood. Some reasons are known with confidence:

1. Parasite species: only *Plasmodium falciparum* causes fatal malaria and a variety of severe disease syndromes. The many deaths worldwide each year (estimated to total between 0.8 and 2 million: WHO, 1993) are nearly all due to this species.
2. Host resistance: innate and acquired mechanisms influence the severity of symptoms, or prevent symptoms entirely (see Chapter 3).
3. Transmission intensity: both the age distribution of disease and the pattern of clinical syndromes in a population differ according to the pattern of transmission, which determines who becomes infected and the way in which specific immunity is acquired (see Chapter 1).
4. Anti-malarial drug use, and the drug-susceptibility of parasites in the locality.

Other possible factors that may influence the nature or severity of malaria disease are still speculative: (i) Parasite 'strain': when *P. falciparum* was inoculated via mosquitoes for the treatment of syphilis, strains of parasite were 'recognized as distinct by their clinical virulence' (Covell and Nicol, 1951). More recently *P. falciparum* isolates from patients with severe malaria have been reported to have characteristics distinguishing them from other isolates, e.g. greater rosetting capacity (Treutiger et al, 1992), greater stimulus to cytokine production by cultured monocytes (Allan et al, 1993: see Chapter 9) or particular in vitro cytoadherence characteristics (Ho et al, 1991). None of these features is reliably associated with 'virulence', however, and the importance of parasite strains in determining disease remains unclear. (ii) Sporozoite inoculum dose: in induced ('therapeutic') malaria, the number of sporozoites inoculated affected neither the incubation period nor the severity of malaria (Yorke and Macfie, 1924). In natural infections sporozoite dose is difficult to measure or estimate (Glynn et al, 1994), so its influence on disease is uncertain.

Baillière's Clinical Infectious Diseases—
Vol. 2, No. 2, July 1995
ISBN 0–7020–1983–6

ASYMPTOMATIC PARASITAEMIA

In endemic areas a large proportion of individuals may be parasitaemic but not sick (see Chapter 3). In such circumstances, defining the spectrum of clinical features attributable to malaria is difficult. A level of parasitaemia (usually 5000–20 000 µl) above which symptoms are likely to be present can be calculated for a given population (Smith et al, 1994); this is useful for epidemiological purposes, but is less helpful clinically.

UNCOMPLICATED MALARIA: THE FEBRILE ILLNESS

Fever is characteristic of all human malarias, and associated symptoms such as headache, myalgia, chills, rigors and sweating (Warrell, 1993) are usual. Symptoms may develop in the classical sequence: cold stage, then hot stage, then sweating. But this progression is often absent. The level of pyrexia tends to be less in *P. malariae* infections than others (Shute, 1952) and rigors are more common in *P. vivax* than *P. falciparum* infections (Covell and Nicol, 1951). Anaemia may develop with heavy or protracted infections with any species of *Plasmodium*, and splenomegaly is usual.

Common reasons for clinical misdiagnosis of uncomplicated malaria

These include:

1. Failure to consider malaria because a travel history is not taken; the history should cover several years. For residents in a malarious country, travel or migration within the country is important if transmission is focal. A very brief visit to an endemic area (e.g. airport touch-down) is sufficient for infection (Conlon et al, 1990). (Because mosquitoes may 'commute' in baggage, malaria is occasionally transmitted in non-malarious countries, usually, but not necessarily, near airports: Castelli et al, 1994.)
2. The belief that malarial fevers always have a characteristic pattern. In fact the classical fever rhythms, tertian (fever spikes on days 1 and 3) and quartan (fever spikes on days 1 and 4) are seldom seen for the first few days of the illness, when pyrexia may be sustained, irregular or quotidian (daily) irrespective of parasite species (Covell and Nicol, 1951).
3. The fact that other symptoms may accompany fever and suggest another diagnosis. Cough and tachypnoea are common in children with malaria, making symptom-based diagnosis unreliable, particularly in distinguishing malaria from acute respiratory infection in malarious areas (Redd et al, 1992; O'Dempsey et al, 1993). Vomiting, diarrhoea, abdominal pain and mild jaundice may each be a presenting feature of malaria suggesting an alternative diagnosis.
4. In an endemic area, assuming a diagnosis of malaria in a febrile patient because malaria is common. Even if parasitaemia is found, an alternative or additional diagnosis may be the cause of illness.

5. Neglect of the incubation period (interval from inoculation to illness); this is at least 7 days in *P. falciparum* malaria, somewhat longer in the other malarias, and sometimes greatly prolonged (months in falciparum, years in other malarias), especially if chemoprophylaxis has been used (Wernsdorfer and McGregor, 1988).
6. Rejection of the diagnosis because of a negative blood film or absence of fever. Symptoms may develop when levels of parasitaemia are too low to detect by microscopy; repeated films may reveal parasites, but treatment on the basis of clinical suspicion is sometimes warranted, especially in patients who have been taking anti-malarial chemoprophylaxis. Fever is irregular or sometimes periodic; a patient may be apyrexial when first seen, and occasionally the temperature may remain normal or low during several days of observation and treatment (Wirima and Harries, 1987).

Failure to diagnose and treat malaria promptly can be disastrous in *P. falciparum* infections because of the risk of progression to severe and complicated disease (Molyneux and Fox, 1993).

DIAGNOSTIC METHODS

Because immunity can affect the clinical manifestations of malaria, diagnosis must always include two questions: is malaria *infection* present? and is malaria responsible for the patient's *illness*?

In endemic populations, parasitaemia is almost universal in some age groups and may be irrelevant to the current illness. The clinician is usually obliged to treat parasites once found, while also considering other possible diagnoses. For research purposes a definition of clinical malaria must be developed, based on symptoms and a minimum density of parasitaemia calculated from surveys of appropriate age groups of the local asymptomatic population (Armstrong-Schellenberg et al, 1994).

In non-immune individuals any parasitaemia is likely to give rise to symptoms, and some subjects develop mild or even severe disease with low, occasionally undetectable, levels of peripheral parasitaemia.

Blood films

The mainstay of diagnosis and still the basis of clinical practice is the stained peripheral blood film. Thin blood films, made as for standard examination of red and white cells (Giemsa or Leishmann stain), allow optimal examination of parasite morphology (WHO, 1991). A thick blood film (a small drop of blood spread evenly over 1 cm^2 of slide, stained with Giemsa) is essential for identifying a low-density parasitaemia and is therefore the most appropriate screening test. Blood films provide the opportunity to identify the *species* of parasite and the *density* of parasitaemia, which should be calculated by counting parasites against white cells (thick film, for low densities) or red cells (thin film, for high densities).

Dipstick antigen detection test

Basing diagnosis on blood films has several major disadvantages in endemic areas: a functioning microscope is needed; staff trained in staining techniques and microscopy must be available; and there is an inevitable delay between the taking of a blood sample and the provision of a result, during which time treatment is commonly dispensed anyway.

Antigen detection is an attractive alternative, and a method—the *Para*Sight®-F Test—recently developed by Becton Dickinson Advanced Diagnostics, is based on detection of *P. falciparum* histidine-rich protein-2 (HRP-2) in a haemolysed blood sample. A dipstick pre-treated with mouse monoclonal antibody to HRP-2 is placed in a drop of the patient's haemolysed blood. HRP-2 on the stick is then detected by a further (rabbit) anti-HRP-2 reagent containing a coloured marker. The test can be taught to village health workers, requires no equipment additional to the test kit, and survives tropical temperatures for at least a year (Shiff et al, 1994). Both the sensitivity and specificity of the method are between 80% and 100% when compared with blood films, being optimal at parasite densities above 60/μl of blood (Beadle et al, 1994).

This test is likely to make an important contribution to malaria diagnosis for both clinical and epidemiological purposes in endemic areas.

Other methods of parasite detection

A number of methods for quick microscopic identification of parasites in peripheral blood films have been described.

In the quantitative buffy coat (QBC) method, whole blood is centrifuged in a microcapillary tube lined with anticoagulant and acridine orange; parasitized erythrocytes have lower density than unparasitized red cells, and concentrate immediately below the buffy coat, where they are spread out against the edge of the tube by a glass float. Parasites and leukocytes take up the dye and can be identified with ultraviolet (UV) light. The method is accurate, much quicker than traditional microscopy, and inexpensive when a simple UV attachment for a standard microscope is used (Spielman and Perrone, 1989).

An alternative method makes use of an interference filter system to detect acridine orange-stained parasites in thick or thin blood films (Kawamoto, 1991; Wongsrichanalai et al, 1992).

Both of these techniques allow quicker screening of blood samples than is possible with traditional blood films, and are particularly useful for excluding the presence of parasites. Both methods rely on microscopy and trained staff and are therefore of limited potential in field settings.

Molecular methods of parasite detection

Many methods for detecting parasite DNA have been described; the general applicability of these methods for clinical purposes is limited by the need for appropriate equipment and expertise. A nested polymerase chain reaction (PCR) for detection of sequences in parasites' small subunit ribo-somal RNA (ssRNA) has made it possible to detect very low levels of infection and differentiate accurately between the four species of human malaria (Snounou et al, 1993).

This technique, while not being appropriate for routine use in the field, may be valuable for screening large numbers of samples in field surveys and in elucidating the epidemiology of different human malarias, especially when these occur concurrently in a single population.

PCR methods of malaria diagnosis are more fully described in Chapter 8.

COMPLICATED *P. FALCIPARUM* MALARIA

In a proportion of cases, *P. falciparum* infection progresses from mild ill-ness to severe or complicated disease. In areas of intense transmission, e.g. many countries in subSaharan Africa, those affected are predominantly (not exclusively) children. In epidemics people of all ages may be affected; in some populations risk is determined by behaviour or activity, e.g. holiday travel, work in forests, migration: in these circumstances adults are at greatest risk.

The definition of 'severe' disease is problematic in a condition with a continuous spectrum of clinical forms. For practical purposes malaria is severe when it is life-threatening. A research definition is recommended by WHO (1990), severity being defined by the presence of any of the following complications: coma, renal failure, severe anaemia, acidosis, respiratory distress syndrome, hypoglycaemia, bleeding, shock, intra-vascular haemolysis. Other features commonly associated with severe disease and which should be included in a practical definition for purposes of clinical management are: lesser degrees of altered consciousness, extreme weakness (prostration), convulsions, jaundice and hyper-parasitaemia (> 2% of red cells parasitized; > 5% in semi-immune popu-lations). The frequency with which various syndromes of severe malaria occur in a population differs according to the local transmission pattern and therefore with the age of people predominantly affected.

SEVERE MALARIA IN CHILDREN IN AREAS WITH INTENSE TRANSMISSION

Severe malaria is a major cause of morbidity, hospital admissions and death (see Chapter 1). In the absence of drug treatment it is thought that about one infection in a hundred may be fatal (Greenwood et al, 1987).

The pattern of severe disease is considerably different from that seen in non-immune adults. In children in high-transmission areas (mainly subSaharan Africa) some of the organ complications characteristic of severe malaria in adults, e.g. renal failure, adult respiratory distress syndrome, bleeding diathesis, are rare.

Five clinical patterns predominate as the presenting syndromes of severe falciparum malaria in African children: severe anaemia, encephalopathy ('cerebral malaria'), acidosis, hypoglycaemia and respiratory distress. These may occur singly or in any combination; hypoglycaemia and acidosis are common (not invariable) components of the cerebral malaria syndrome, and respiratory distress is frequently (not always) associated with acidosis. In reported subSaharan African studies, severe anaemia has a peak incidence at around 2 years of age (Brewster, 1992), while the median age for cerebral malaria is about 3 years (Molyneux et al, 1989b; Marsh et al, 1995). Two studies have compared disease patterns between areas with intense transmission (e.g. 30–300 infective mosquito bites/year) and areas with less transmission (1–10 bites/year, with seasonal fluctuations: Slutsker et al, 1994; Snow et al, 1994): in both studies, severe anaemia was the predominating complication in the population subjected to higher-intensity transmission, while cerebral malaria was more common in the areas of less intense transmission. Therefore, severe malaria affected children of a younger age, on average, in the areas with more intense transmission.

Severe anaemia in children

In holoendemic areas *P. falciparum* is the predominant cause of anaemia, and severe anaemia is a common cause of hospital admission. Among children admitted to hospital with haemoglobin concentrations below 5.1 g/dl, case fatality is 6–18%, the case fatality being significantly greater among children with respiratory distress than among those without (Lackritz et al, 1992). Case fatality is greatest in infants and progressively less with increasing age (Brewster, 1992). Death may be due to cardiac failure (Newton et al, 1992; Craighead and Knowles, 1993) or to other complications of malaria. It seems likely that anaemia, whatever the cause, may alter the child's susceptibility to infections, especially pneumonia; pallor suggesting anaemia was present in 20% of fatal and 3% of non-fatal respiratory infections among children in rural Tanzania (Mtango et al, 1989).

Mortality in the community due to severe malarial anaemia is difficult to estimate (Snow et al, 1992), but is likely to be considerable. Effective clearance of parasitaemia appears to improve the resolution of anaemia (Bloland et al, 1992), and increasing parasite drug resistance in a population may therefore lead to an increase in the prevalence of anaemia.

Cerebral malaria (CM) in children

This syndrome, characterized by altered consciousness and convulsions, is probably the commonest mode of death due to malaria in children. The mean age of affected children is usually about 3 years. A notable feature is the rapidity of onset of the syndrome: the mean interval between the first symptom (usually feverishness) and loss of consciousness is less than 48 hours, and in many cases less than 24 hours (Molyneux et al, 1989b).

The mortality of cerebral malaria in the absence of treatment is not known; hospital mortality in children admitted with unrousable coma is 15–30% (see *Prognostic indicators in paediatric cerebral malaria*, on page 281).

Altered consciousness

This may be of any degree. In children who recover, the duration of coma after the start of treatment is on average 18–36 hours, a figure which may be affected by the drug treatment used (Taylor et al, 1993b). It is traditional to attempt to measure the depth of coma with a coma score (see Table 1), of which several versions suitable for children have been developed (Reilly et al, 1988; Molyneux et al, 1989b). None of these scoring systems is strictly a measure of consciousness; each involves assessment of associated motor or sensory capabilities. A score is valuable for monitoring progress and for defining categories of disease severity.

Table 1. A coma score for children.

Clinical measurement	Score
Best motor response:	
Localizes painful stimulus[a]	2
Withdraws limb from painful stimulus[b]	1
No response or inappropriate response	0
Best verbal response:	
Cries or speaks appropriately with stimulus[a]	2
Moan or abnormal cry with stimulus[a]	1
No vocal response to painful stimulus	0
Eye movement:	
Watches or follows (e.g. mother's face)	1
Fails to watch or follow	0
To obtain coma score, add scores for each section	

After Molyneux et al (1989b).
This score is not suitable for children under the age of 6 months.
[a] Pressure on sternum with blunt end of pencil.
[b] Pressure with horizontal pencil on nailbed

The most profoundly comatose patients lose brain stem reflexes, indicated by abnormal caloric and 'doll's eye' tests. Corneal and rarely pupillary responses are absent in some cases.

Convulsions

These occur in 60–80% of children with CM. Some seizure activity may be identifiable by electro-encephalography in children without clinically detectable convulsions (J. Crawley et al, unpublished data). Fits may be focal or generalized or both. In some children convulsions are associated with a recognized cause, such as hypoglycaemia or hyperpyrexia. In others no cause other than malaria can be identified. Febrile convulsions may occur in any child with fever; consciousness is usually regained within a few minutes of a febrile convulsion, but coma persists if malaria is the cause. There is some evidence that malaria-associated convulsions, even if apparently 'febrile' in character (i.e. followed by rapid regaining of consciousness), differ from febrile convulsions associated with other causes of fever; convulsions are more common in malaria than other fevers and are more likely to be complex (C. Waruiru, personal communication).

Convulsions may be single or recurrent, before or during treatment. It may be difficult to decide clinically whether motor abnormalities, e.g. posturing of limbs, conjugate deviation of eyes, are in fact convulsive in nature. Convulsions may be complicated by anoxia or by aspiration pneumonia, which in some patients is the cause of death.

Abnormalities of tone and posture

A child with CM may be motionless and hypotonic, or have a generalized increase of muscle tone, with the posture of decerebrate or decorticate rigidity or opisthotonos (Figure 1). Commonly posturing is episodic, or there may be periodic exacerbations of its severity, with new positions of limbs or trunk sustained for periods of a few seconds, repeated at intervals. Conjugate deviation of the eyes, with or without nystagmus, is often present and may be episodic.

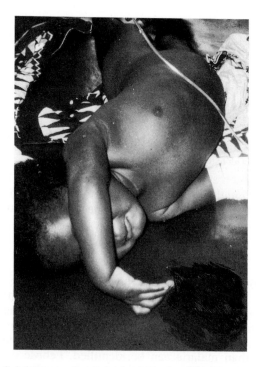

Figure 1. Opisthotonus and posturing in a Malawian child with cerebral malaria.

Abnormalities of breathing

Fever may cause tachypnoea, but additional respiratory features are common in children with CM. Acidosis may be accompanied by deep breathing. Cheyne–Stokes or other irregular breathing patterns may be present in the profoundly unconscious. Tachypnoea is exacerbated in the presence of aspiration pneumonia, in profound anaemia, and in pulmonary oedema which may result from over-infusion of fluids.

Respiratory distress, with or without acidosis, is also a manifestation of severe malaria in the conscious child (Marsh et al, 1995).

Hypoglycaemia

About one third of children admitted to hospital with CM and unrousable coma are hypoglycaemic (plasma glucose < 2.2 mmol/l: White et al, 1987; Taylor et al, 1988; Phillips, 1989). Hypoglycaemia cannot be diagnosed by clinical examination alone, since the clinical features of hypoglycaemia are similar to those of CM. In a few cases correction of hypoglycaemia results in improvement or recovery of consciousness, but in the majority there is no such effect, suggesting that hypoglycaemia alone is not the cause of coma. Hypoglycaemia is accompanied by appropriately low plasma insulin concentrations, and may recur during treatment even if glucose supplements are maintained. Children with hypoglycaemia tend to be younger and are more likely to be profoundly unconscious, convulsing, acidotic and hyperparasitaemic than others, and have an increased risk of prolonged coma, sequelae and death (Taylor et al, 1988).

Abnormalities of optic fundi

Retinal haemorrhages (both dot and blot varieties, some with white centres) are commonly found in children with CM (Davis et al, 1982; Lewallen et al, 1993). Other lesions of the optic fundi recently described are macular oedema, extramacular oedema and papilloedema (S. Lewallen et al, unpublished data), the latter sign being present in 11% of 141 Malawian children with unrousable coma due to CM. In this study, only papilloedema was significantly associated with a high cerebrospinal fluid opening pressure, and papilloedema and extramacular oedema were independently predictive of a fatal outcome.

Raised intracranial pressure

Most children with CM have opening pressures at lumbar puncture that are above the range usually considered normal. In one study, progressive brain stem dysfunction preceding death was considered as a possible indicator of central cerebral herniation, and the potential danger of lumbar puncture in CM was discussed (Newton et al, 1991). When mean opening pressures in 26 fatal and 70 non-fatal cases in Malawi, The Gambia and Thailand were compared, no difference was found (Kwiatkowski et al, 1991; Waller et al,

1991; White, 1991), and estimated cerebral perfusion pressures were above 30 mmHg in nearly all cases. Single measurements of intracranial pressure do not accurately predict maximum or sustained levels, and intracranial pressures recorded by an implanted transducer in children with CM show great fluctuations over time (Newton et al, 1994). Whether raised intracranial pressure contributes to coma or death in some patients can only be established by trials of interventions against the possible pathogenetic mechanisms.

Acidosis

Children with CM may be severely acidotic (Taylor et al, 1993a; Krishna et al, 1994), and acidosis may also complicate severe non-cerebral malaria (Marsh et al, 1995). In some cases metabolic acidosis is compensated by increased ventilation; in others there is incomplete respiratory compensation and acidaemia results (Taylor et al, 1993a). There are high concentrations of lactate in plasma and cerebrospinal fluid (White et al, 1987; Taylor et al, 1988). Acidaemia is rapidly corrected by effective antiparasitic treatment and fluid and glucose replacement, except in patients proceeding to a fatal outcome, in whom raised lactate levels persist (Krishna et al, 1994).

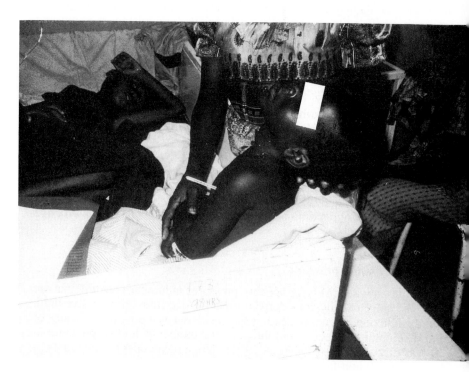

Figure 2. Hypotonia in a Malawian child 2 days after recovery of consciousness in cerebral malaria.

Neurological sequelae

Most children who survive CM appear to make a complete recovery. Occasionally a child remains severely hypotonic for a few days after recovery of consciousness (Figure 2). However, about 10% are left with neurological sequelae identifiable by routine clinical examination (Molyneux et al, 1989b; Brewster et al, 1990; Bondi, 1992). Sequelae that have been described include hemiparesis, cerebellar ataxia, blindness, deafness, generalized spasticity, aphasia, mental retardation and ocular palsies (Figure 3). A child's neurological status may improve or resolve over subsequent months, but about 50% of sequelae persist. Defects suggestive of cerebral infarction can be seen in CAT-scans of the brain in some children with sequelae (Newton et al, 1994). It seems likely that a proportion of children without gross neurological impairment may have more subtle forms of brain damage affecting motor or learning abilities; this possibility is being investigated in current field studies in The Gambia and Kenya.

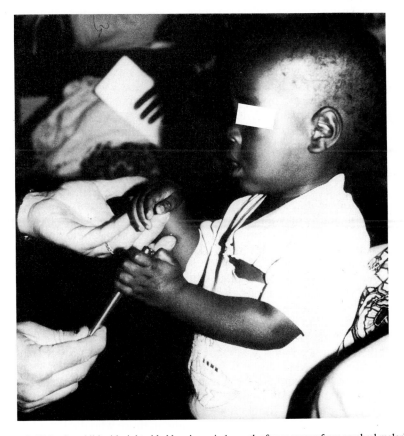

Figure 3. Malawian child with right-sided hemiparesis 1 month after recovery from cerebral malaria.

Prognostic indicators in paediatric cerebral malaria

A number of studies have now been completed comparing clinical features between children with CM who survive and those who do not (Molyneux et al, 1989b). The strongest predictors of death are profound coma, acidosis and hypoglycaemia. Other presenting features that have been found to be associated with a fatal outcome are: very high parasite density, predominance of large ring-stage parasites in the peripheral blood (Silamut and White, 1993), witnessed or repeated convulsions, papilloedema and/or extramacular retinal oedema (Lewallen et al, 1993), plasma tumour necrosis factor concentration (Grau et al, 1989; Kwiatkowski et al, 1990) and biochemical evidence of impaired hepatic or renal function (Sowumni, personal communication). Prognostic indicators for sequelae are similar to those that are associated with death.

Muscle abnormalities in severe malaria in children

Myalgia and muscular weakness are common symptoms in both mild and severe malaria (Warrell, 1993). In some cases weakness is profound, and severe hypotonia may persist for a period of days after recovery of consciousness in patients with cerebral malaria (unpublished data). Serum myoglobin and creatine kinase levels are raised in the majority of children with cerebral malaria and in a minority of patients with less severe disease (Miller et al, 1989). A muscle biopsy in a man aged 17 years with malaria, severe muscle pain and myoglobinuria showed necrosis and fragmentation of myofibrils (De Silva et al, 1988).

COMPLICATED *P. FALCIPARUM* MALARIA IN ADULTS

In populations not continuously exposed to *P. falciparum* in childhood, infections in adults may progress to severe disease. The pattern of complicated disease differs in several respects from that seen in children. Organ complications such as acute renal failure and adult respiratory distress syndrome are more likely to develop in adults, sometimes in association with altered consciousness but often in the absence of cerebral disease. Any or all of the complications listed as defining severe malaria (see *Complicated* P. Falciparum *malaria*, on page 275), may occur in any combination; in the most severely ill, many organs or systems tend to be affected concurrently.

Delay in diagnosis and treatment may increase the likelihood of the development of severe disease. In Britain in 1991–1993 there were 27 deaths from malaria; among these individuals the median interval between first symptom and diagnosis was 5 days (range 1–35: Malaria Reference Laboratory, London). Although there was a similar delay in non-fatal malaria, it is likely that more prompt therapy in those who died would have reduced the case fatality.

Cerebral malaria (CM) in adults

The features described in children, above, are all commonly seen in adults, and the hospital case-fatality rate is similar. Notable differences between CM in adults and CM in children are:

1. The interval between first symptom and onset of coma is longer on average in adults.
2. The mean interval between the start of treatment and recovery of consciousness is also longer in adults.
3. Parasite densities tend to be higher in children than adults.
4. Other organ complications are frequently associated with CM in adults but not in children.
5. Cerebrospinal fluid opening pressures are usually within the normal range in adults but are usually high in children.
6. Hypoglycaemia as a presenting feature is more common in children.
7. Neurological sequelae are more frequently seen in children than adults (WHO, 1990).

The comatose adult may exhibit hypertonicity, posturing, extensor plantar responses, conjugate gaze deviation, nystagmus and primitive reflexes (grasp, palmar-mental, pouting: Warrell et al, 1982). Papilloedema is rare but retinal haemorrhages are common. Retinal haemorrhages are more frequently seen in CM than in non-cerebral malaria, but among CM patients they are not significantly associated with fatal disease (Looareesuwan et al, 1983).

In patients with unrousable coma who survive, the mean time from the start of treatment until recovery of consciousness is about 42 hours (Warrell et al, 1982). Convulsions are common both before and during treatment (White et al, 1988); as in children, these may take a variety of forms from focal to grand-mal seizures.

Spinal fluid opening pressures at the start of treatment range from 40 to 320 mm csf (cerebrospinal fluid), the mean and range being similar in those who die and those who recover (White, 1986).

Renal failure

Acute renal failure (ARF) due to acute tubular necrosis is a common component of the severe malaria syndrome in adults. This complication developed in 30% of 346 adults with severe malaria in a Vietnamese hospital in 1988 (Trang et al, 1992). Risk factors for the development of renal failure include hyperparasitaemia, shock, and severe intravascular haemolysis. Delayed treatment of malaria and late or inadequate correction of volume depletion are probable contributing factors in some cases. Jaundice commonly accompanies renal failure, and pulmonary and/or cerebral complications of malaria are frequently present, especially in fatal cases (Stone et al, 1972; Trang et al, 1992). In some reported series oliguria (24-hour urine volume < 400 ml/day, unresponsive to fluid replacement) is included in the definition of ARF; patients may be oliguric or anuric, the latter having a worse prognosis. It seems clear, however, that oliguria is not invariable in ARF, and some patients may even be polyuric (Phillips et al, 1984).

The reversibility of the renal lesion has been well shown by the reduction in mortality achieved by introducing peritoneal or haemo-dialysis, from 50% to 14% in a study in Thailand (Stone et al, 1972) and from 75% to 26% in a hospital in Vietnam (Trang et al, 1992). The interval between the start of dialysis and recovery of renal function is usually a few days, but occasionally up to 4 weeks (Indrapasit et al, 1988). Death may be due to complications of renal failure, including cardiac arrest due to hyperkalaemia, pulmonary oedema and haemorrhage, or to concomitant bacteraemia, cerebral malaria or respiratory distress syndrome.

Lesser degrees of renal 'dysfunction' without ARF may be detected biochemically in patients with severe malaria, including children, and are associated with severity of disease and poor prognosis.

Adult respiratory distress syndrome (ARDS)

Patients with or without cerebral complications may develop a pulmonary syndrome characterized by tachypnoea, hypoxia, and perihilar or widespread shadowing on chest X-ray (Figure 4) (Brooks et al, 1968). Clinically the distinction must be made between pulmonary oedema, which may result from excessive fluid infusion (especially in the presence of acute renal failure) and ARDS (James, 1985). Records of a large positive fluid

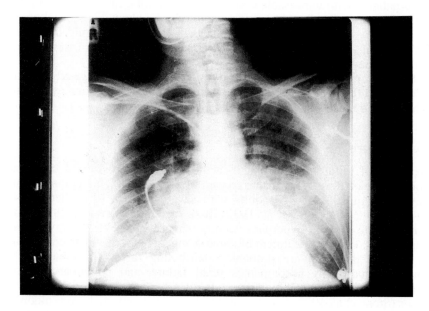

Figure 4. Chest radiograph in a British adult with respiratory distress syndrome due to *P. falciparum* infection.

balance and the presence of a raised central venous pressure suggest a diagnosis of pulmonary oedema; the two conditions are best distinguished by measuring the pulmonary artery wedge pressure, which is high in pulmonary oedema but normal in ARDS. Since both ARDS and pulmonary oedema are common in patients with ARF, the two forms of pulmonary complication may coexist in the same patient.

ARDS is a grave complication with a high mortality (Brooks et al, 1968), especially if facilities for intensive care, including artificial ventilation, are not available.

Bronchopneumonia may complicate cerebral malaria, especially in patients who have required intubation and assisted ventilation.

Disseminated intravascular coagulation (DIC)

Thrombocytopenia is usual in both mild and severe falciparum malaria; this probably results from reduced platelet lifespan (Horstmann et al, 1981), antibody-mediated platelet aggregation (Mohanty et al, 1988) and possibly platelet sequestration. Evidence of minor degrees of DIC can be found in many patients with severe malaria, but this is rarely accompanied by prolonged bleeding. Antithrombin III concentrations are reduced (Phillips et al, 1986). Identifying DIC can be obscured by the fact that fibrinogen levels increase as part of the acute phase response (Pukrittayakamee et al, 1989). In about 5% of patients with complicated malaria, overt spontaneous bleeding occurs requiring replacement therapy (Phillips et al, 1986). The risk of bleeding may be exacerbated in the presence of renal failure and sepsis.

Shock

Hypotension and impaired peripheral perfusion occur in some adults with severe malaria. In some instances, as in 10 out of 175 Thai patients with cerebral malaria, shock is accompanied by, and probably attributable to, bacteraemia (Warrell et al, 1982). Indwelling urinary or vascular catheters increase the risk of bloodborne infection. The presence of shock increases the risk of acute tubular necrosis.

Disturbances of liver and gastrointestinal tract

Minor degrees of jaundice are frequently seen in patients with falciparum malaria, and malaria may be misdiagnosed as viral hepatitis with disastrous consequences. In malaria both hepatocellular dysfunction and haemolysis may contribute to jaundice. Slight elevations of plasma concentrations of liver enzymes are common, but increases of the degree usual in viral hepatitis are not found. Frank hepatic failure does not occur.

Hepatic blood flow is decreased in severe malaria in association with a decrease in splanchnic blood flow and impairment of gut absorptive function (Molyneux et al, 1989a; Pukrittayakamee et al, 1992). Impaired caffeine clearance in patients with severe malaria and jaundice indicates reduced hepatocellular microsomal function (Wilairatana et al, 1994). Diarrhoea is sometimes a symptom of malaria but is rarely severe. Occasionally upper gastrointestinal haemorrhage complicates severe malaria, exacerbated by DIC and intense sequestration of parasitized erythrocytes in gut microvasculature (unpublished data).

Hypoglycaemia

This may complicate untreated malaria in adults (Migasena, 1983; Kiire, 1986), especially in pregnancy; this complication is less common than it is in children. Hypoglycaemia may develop as a result of quinine-induced hyperinsulinaemia, usually after quinine has been administered over a few days; pregnant women are particularly susceptible to this effect of quinine (White et al, 1983).

Cardiac effects

Although sequestration of parasitized erythrocytes is sometimes prominent in myocardial tissue, abnormalities of cardiac function or rhythm are rare in malaria unless there is profound anaemia, drug toxicity or hyperkalaemia (in renal failure; Trang et al, 1992). In cerebral malaria in both children and adults death is seldom attributable to cardiac arrest, and the heart may continue to beat after spontaneous breathing has stopped (unpublished data).

Inappropriate secretion of anti-diuretic hormone (ADH)

Hyponatraemia is a common finding in severe malaria (Miller et al, 1967). Sometimes this can be attributed to excessive intake or infusion of hypo-tonic fluid, either in the presence of renal impairment or after a period of prolonged salt loss through sweating (Fryatt et al, 1989). In other cases there is evidence of inappropriate secretion of ADH, as in a recent series of 17 consecutive adult admissions for severe malaria: 13 of the patients were hyponatraemic, 6 of these having features of inappropriate ADH secretion, with high urine sodium concentrations, low serum osmolality and inappro-priately high plasma ADH concentrations (Holst et al, 1994).

MALARIA AND PREGNANCY

The clinical impact of malaria differs according to the level of endemicity. Most available data concern *P. falciparum* infections.

In *P. falciparum* holoendemic areas

Here, pregnant women are more likely to be parasitaemic than non-pregnant women of the same age, and parasite counts tend to be higher in pregnancy; these differences are greatest in the second trimester and in primigravidae (Brabin, 1983; McGregor, 1984). There is no convincing evidence that pregnant women suffer more symptomatic malaria than non-pregnant women; malarial infection and pregnancy are separate causes of anaemia, and it is not clear whether the two occurring together are potentiating or merely additive. Maternal and placental malaria are associated with low birth weight in the babies of primigravidae (Brabin, 1983; McGregor et al, 1983), this being mainly due to growth retardation rather than prematurity. One study (Nyirjesy et al, 1993) has reported an increased perinatal death rate in babies born to mothers with malaria, but this has not been the case in other studies. Malaria-associated low birth weight carries an increased risk of death in infancy (R. Steketee, personal communication).

In areas of low or unstable transmission

Here, pregnant women suffer more severe disease than non-pregnant women when infected with *P. falciparum* (Subramanian et al, 1992; Nosten et al, 1994). In pregnancy women are particularly prone to hypoglycaemia, whether due to malaria or to quinine therapy (White et al, 1983; Looareesuwan et al, 1985). There is an increased risk of fetal loss, intrauterine death and neonatal death and increased maternal mortality.

CONGENITAL MALARIA

In holoendemic areas *P. falciparum* may occasionally be found in umbilical venous blood (Nyirjesy et al, 1993); fewer parasites are found in peripheral blood, and within 24–48 hours these have disappeared. Symptomatic malarial illness in neonates is rare. It is likely that when malaria develops in infancy it is due to newly acquired rather than trans-placental infection (McGregor, 1984).

   In areas of low transmission or in non-immunes, malaria in the mother at term may be followed by 'congenital malaria' in the infant. The species of *Plasmodium* causing congenital infection is largely determined by circumstances and geographical setting: *P. falciparum* predominated in one review (Hulbert, 1992), *P. vivax* in another (Covell, 1950). Symptoms begin to appear between 2 weeks and 2 months of age and consist of fever and failure to feed; hepatosplenomegaly and anaemia are usual.

CHRONIC COMPLICATIONS OF MALARIA

Hyperreactive malarial splenomegaly

In populations subjected to intense transmission of *P. falciparum*, some individuals develop massive enlargement of the spleen which cannot be attributed to any cause other than frequent previous malaria infections. In many cases plasma total IgM concentration is raised and hepatic sinusoids are infiltrated with lymphocytes, but neither of these features is invariable.

Young adults are most frequently affected, women more often than men. In most populations this syndrome is uncommon, but in one community in Papua New Guinea, 60% of adults were affected (Crane, 1986), and in a hospital antenatal department in Ghana 5–8% of pregnant women had clinical problems related to massive splenomegaly (Bates, 1991). The very large spleen may cause mechanical symptoms, anaemia and thrombocytopenia ('hypersplenism'), and is susceptible to injury. Long-term antimalarial therapy leads to gradual resolution.

The pathogenesis of hyperreactive malarial splenomegaly is discussed in Chapter 2.

Nephrotic syndrome of *P. malariae* infection

P. malariae has been identified as a possible cause of nephrotic syndrome in some populations (Gilles and Hendrickse, 1963). The syndrome is associated with *P. malariae* parasitaemia and became rare when antimalarial measures were introduced, for example in Sierra Leone and Guyana (Kibukamusoke, 1973). The complication affects only a minority of infected individuals, mainly children, and tends to run a relentless course unresponsive to corticosteroid or anti-malarial therapy, although some patients may benefit partially from cytotoxic drugs. The association between quartan malaria and nephrotic syndrome has not been found in all populations with endemic *P. malariae* transmission.

The immunological basis of malarial nephropathy is discussed in Chapter 2.

Burkitt's lymphoma

Malaria may play a part in the aetiology of this common tumour, which occurs with much greater frequency in subSaharan Africa and Papua New Guinea than in other parts of the world. In both regions the distribution of Burkitt's lymphoma parallels that of hyperendemic *P. falciparum* malaria. The association of Burkitt's lymphoma with Epstein–Barr virus infection is well established; malaria may be responsible for altering the host's response to the virus in some individuals, leading to neoplastic change (Burkitt, 1969; Whittle et al, 1984). The current understanding of possible mechanisms of this interaction is discussed in Chapter 2.

SUMMARY

The clinical effects of malarial infection range from none to fatal disease, depending on parasitic, host and environmental factors. In a non-immune individual any *P. falciparum* infection must be regarded as potentially serious and treated urgently. Early symptoms may be misleading, especially if exposure history is neglected; delayed recognition may be disastrous. Thick and thin blood films are still the mainstay of diagnosis. In endemic areas young children suffer most of the severe illness from

P. falciparum infections, and in first pregnancy susceptibility is increased and intra-uterine growth may be impaired. Malaria is a major cause of death in young children in endemic areas, and some of those who survive severe illness have neurological sequelae. In non-immune adults, untreated *P. falciparum* infection may cause a variety of potentially fatal organ complications. Malaria continues to be an important risk for the unprotected traveller to areas where the parasite is transmitted.

REFERENCES

Allan RJ, Rowe A & Kwiatkowski D (1993) *Plasmodium falciparum* varies in its ability to induce tumor necrosis factor. *Infection and Immunology* **61**: 4772–4776.

Armstrong-Schellenberg JRM, Smith T, Alonso PL & Hayes RJ (1994) What is clinical malaria? Finding case definitions for field research in highly endemic areas. *Parasitology Today* **10**: 439–442.

Bates I (1991) Hyperreactive malarial splenomegaly in pregnancy. *Tropical Doctor* **21**: 101–103.

Beadle C, Long GW, Weiss WR et al (1994) Diagnosis of malaria by detection of *Plasmodium falciparum* HRP-2 antigen with a rapid dipstick antigen-capture assay. *Lancet* **334**: 564–568.

Bloland PB, Lackritz EM, Kazembe PN et al (1992) Beyond chloroquine: implications of drug resistance for evaluating malaria therapy efficacy and treatment policy in Africa. *Journal of Infectious Diseases* **167**: 932–937.

Bondi FS (1992) The incidence and outcome of neurological abnormalities in childhood cerebral malaria: a long-term follow-up of 62 survivors. *Transactions of the Royal Society of Tropical Medicine and Hygiene* **86**: 17–19.

Brabin BJ (1983) An analysis of malaria in pregnancy in Africa. *Bulletin of the World Health Organization* **61**: 1005–1016.

Brewster DR, Kwiatkowski D & White NJ (1990) Neurological sequelae of cerebral malaria in children. *Lancet* **336**: 1039–1043.

Brewster DR (1992) Blood transfusions for severe anaemia in African children. *Lancet* **340**: 917 (letter).

Brooks MH, Kiel FW, Sheehy TW & Barry KG (1968) Acute pulmonary edema in falciparum malaria. *New England Journal of Medicine* **279(14)**: 732–737.

Burkitt D (1969) Aetiology of Burkitt's lymphoma—an alternative hypothesis to a vectored virus. *Journal of the National Cancer Institute* **42**: 19–28.

Castelli F, Cabona MG, Brunori A & Carosi G (1994) Imported mosquito: an uninvited guest. *American Journal of Tropical Medicine and Hygiene* **50(5)**: 548–549.

Conlon CP, Berendt AR, Dawson K & Peto TEA (1990) Runway malaria. *Lancet* **335**: 472–473.

Covell G (1950) Congenital malaria. *Tropical Diseases Bulletin* **47(12)**: 1147–1167.

Covell G & Nicol WD (1951) Clinical, chemotherapeutic and immunological studies on induced malaria. *British Medical Bulletin* **8(1)**: 51–55.

Craighead IB & Knowles JK (1993) Prevention of transfusion-associated HIV transmission with the use of a transfusion protocol for under 5s. *Tropical Doctor* **23**: 59–61.

Crane GG (1986) Hyperreactive malarious splenomegaly (tropical splenomegaly syndrome). *Parasitology Today* **2**: 4–9.

Davis MW, Vaterlaws AL, Simes J & Torzillo P (1982) Retinopathy in malaria. *Papua New Guinea Medical Journal* **25**: 19–22.

De Silva HJ, Goonetilleke AKE, Senaratna N et al (1988) Skeletal muscle necrosis in severe falciparum malaria *British Medical Journal* **296**: 1039.

Fryatt RJ, Teng JD, Harries AD et al (1989) Plasma and urine electrolyte concentrations and vasopressin levels in patients admitted to hospital for falciparum malaria. *Tropical and Geographical Medicine* **41**: 57–60.

Gilles HM & Hendrickse RG (1963) Nephrosis in Nigerian children: role of *Plasmodium malariae* and effect of antimalarial treatment. *British Medical Journal* **2**: 27–31.

Glynn JR, Lines J & Bradley DJ (1994) Impregnated bednets and the dose-severity relationship in malaria. *Parasitology Today* **10(7)**: 279–281.

Grau GE, Taylor TE, Molyneux ME et al (1989) Tumor necrosis factor and disease severity in children with falciparum malaria. *New England Journal of Medicine* **302**: 1586–1591.

Greenwood BM, Greenwood AM, Bradley AH et al (1987) Death in infancy and early childhood in a well-vaccinated rural West African population. *Annals of Tropical Paediatrics* **7**: 91–99.

Ho M, Singh B, Looareesuwan S et al (1991) Clinical correlates of in vitro *Plasmodium falciparum* cytoadherence. *Infection and Immunology* **59**: 873–878.

Holst FGE, Hemmer CJ, Kern P & Manfred D (1994) Inappropriate secretion of antidiuretic hormone and hyponatremia in severe falciparum malaria. *American Journal of Tropical Medicine and Hygiene* **50(5)**: 602–607.

Horstmann RD, Dietrich M, Bienzle U & Rasche H (1981) Malaria-induced thrombocytopenia. *Blut* **42**: 157–164.

Hulbert TV (1992) Congenital malaria in the United States: report of a case and review. *Clinical Infectious Diseases* **14**: 922–926.

Indrapasit S, Charoenpan P, Suvachittanont O et al (1988) Continuous peritoneal dialysis in acute renal failure from severe falciparum malaria. *Clinical Nephrology* **29**: 127–143.

James MFM (1985) Pulmonary damage associated with falciparum malaria: a report of ten cases. *Annals of Tropical Medicine and Parasitology* **79(2)**: 123–138.

Kawamoto F (1991) Rapid detection of *Plasmodium* by a new 'thick smear' method using transmission fluorescence microscopy: direct staining with acridine orange. *Journal of Protozoology Research* **1**: 27–34.

Kibukamusoku JW (1973) *Nephrotic Syndrome of Quartan Malaria*. London: Edward Arnold.

Kiire CF (1986) Hypoglycaemia and cerebral malaria. *Postgraduate Medical Journal* **62**: 401–402.

Krishna S, Waller DW, ter Kuile F et al (1994) Lactic acidosis and hypoglycaemia in children with severe malaria: pathophysiological and prognostic significance. *Transactions of the Royal Society of Tropical Medicine and Hygiene* **88**: 67–73.

Kwiatkowski D, Hill AVS, Sambou I et al (1990) TNF concentration in fatal cerebral, non-fatal cerebral and uncomplicated *P. falciparum* malaria. *Lancet* **336**: 1201–1205.

Kwiatkowski D, Molyneux M, Taylor T et al (1991) Cerebral malaria. *Lancet* **337**: 1281–1282.

Lackritz EM, Campbell CC, Ruebush TK et al (1992) Effect of blood transfusion on survival among children in a Kenyan hospital. *Lancet* **340**: 524–528.

Lewallen S, Taylor TE, Molyneux ME et al (1993) Ocular fundus findings in Malawian children with cerebral malaria. *Ophthalmology* **100**: 857–861.

Looareesuwan S, Warrell DA, White NJ et al (1983) Retinal haemorrhage, a common sign of prognostic significance in cerebral malaria. *American Journal of Tropical Medicine and Hygiene* **32**: 911–915.

Looareesuwan S, Phillips RE, White NJ et al (1985) Quinine and severe falciparum malaria in late pregnancy. *Lancet* **2**: 4–8.

Marsh K, Forster D, Wariuru C et al (1995) Indicators of life-threatening malaria in African children: clinical spectrum and simplified prognostic criteria. *New England Journal of Medicine* **332**: 1399–1404.

McGregor IA (1984) Epidemiology, malaria and pregnancy. *American Journal of Tropical Medicine and Hygiene* **33(4)**: 517–525.

McGregor IA, Wilson ME & Billewicz WZ (1983) Malaria infection of the placenta in The Gambia, West Africa; its incidence and relationship to stillbirth, birthweight and placental weight. *Transactions of the Royal Society of Tropical Medicine and Hygiene* **77**: 232–244.

Migasena S (1983) Hypoglycaemia in falciparum malaria. *Annals of Tropical Medicine and Parasitology* **77(3)**: 323–324.

Miller KD, White NJ, Lott JA et al (1989) Biochemical evidence of muscle injury in African children with severe malaria. *Journal of Infectious Diseases* **159**: 139–142.

Miller LH, Makaranond P, Sitprifa V et al (1967) Hyponatraemia in malaria. *Annals of Tropical Medicine and Parasitology* **61**: 265–269.

Mohanty D, Marwaha N, Ghosh K et al (1988) Functional and unstructural changes of platelets in malaria infection. *Transactions of the Royal Society of Tropical Medicine and Hygiene* **82**: 369–375.

Molyneux ME & Fox R (1993) Diagnosis and treatment of malaria in Britain. *British Medical Journal* **306**: 1175–1180.

Molyneux ME, Looareesuwan S, Menzies IS et al (1989a) Reduced hepatic blood flow and intestinal malabsorption in severe falciparum malaria. *American Journal of Tropical Medicine and Hygiene* **80(5)**: 470–476.

Molyneux ME, Taylor TE, Wirima JJ & Borgstein A (1989b) Clinical features and prognostic indicators in paediatric cerebral malaria: a study of 131 comatose Malawian children. *Quarterly Journal of Medicine* **71**: 441–459.

Mtango FDE, Neuvians D & Korte R (1989) Magnitude, presentation, management and outcome of acute respiratory infections in children under the age of five in hospitals and rural health centres in Tanzania. *Tropical Medicine and Parasitology* **40**: 97–102.

Newton CRJC, Kirkham FJ, Winstanley PA et al (1991) Intracranial pressure in African children with cerebral malaria. *Lancet* **337**: 573–576.

Newton CRJC, Marsh K, Peshu N & Mwangi I (1992) Blood transfusion for severe anaemia in African children. *Lancet* **340**: 917–918 (letter).

Newton CRJC, Peshu N, Kendall B et al (1994) Brain swelling and ischaemia in Kenyans with cerebral malaria. *Archives of Diseases in Children* **70**: 281–287.

Nosten F, ter Kuile F, Maelankiri L et al (1994) Mefloquine prophylaxis prevents malaria during pregnancy: a double-blind, placebo-controlled study. *Journal of Infectious Diseases* **169**: 595–603.

Nyirjesy P, Kavasya T, Axelrod P & Fischer PR (1993) Malaria during pregnancy: neonatal morbidity and mortality and the efficacy of chloroquine chemoprophylaxis. *Clinical Infectious Diseases* **16**: 127–132.

O'Dempsey TJD, McArdle TF, Laurence BE et al (1993) Overlap in the clinical features of pneumonia and malaria in African children. *Transactions of the Royal Society of Tropical Medicine and Hygiene* **87**: 662–665.

Phillips RE (1989) Hypoglycaemia is an important complication of falciparum malaria. *Quarterly Journal of Medicine* **71(266)**: 477–483.

Phillips RE, White NJ, Looareesuwan S et al (1984) Acute renal failure in falciparum malaria in eastern Thailand: successful use of peritoneal dialysis. *Proceedings of the XI International Congress for Tropical Medicine and Malaria*, 6–11 September, Calgary, Canada.

Phillips RE, Looareesuwan S, Warrell DA et al (1986) The importance of anaemia in cerebral and uncomplicated falciparum malaria: role of complications, dyserythropoiesis and iron sequestration. *Quarterly Journal of Medicine* **58**: 305–323.

Pukrittayakamee S, White NJ, Clemens R et al (1989) Activation of the coagulation cascade in falciparum malaria. *Transactions of the Royal Society of Tropical Medicine and Hygiene* **83**: 761–766.

Pukrittayakamee S, White NJ, Davis TME et al (1992) Hepatic blood flow and metabolism in severe falciparum malaria: clearance of intravenous administered galactose. *Clinical Science* **82**: 63–70.

Redd SC, Bloland PB, Kazwembe PN et al (1992) Usefulness of clinical case definitions in guiding therapy for African children with malaria or pneumonia. *Lancet* **340**: 1140–1143.

Reilly PL, Simpson DA, Sprod R & Thomas L (1988) Assessing the conscious level in infants and young children: a paediatric version of the Glasgow coma scale. *Childhood Nervous System* **4**: 30–33.

Shiff CJ, Minjas J & Premji Z (1994) The *ParaSight*®-F test: a simple rapid manual dipstick test to detect *Plasmodium falciparum* infection. *Parasitology Today* **10**: 494–495.

Shute PG (1952) Malarial fever therapy. *Lancet* **263**: 333–336.

Silamut K & White NJ (1993) Relation of the stage of parasite development in the peripheral blood to prognosis in severe falciparum malaria. *Transactions of the Royal Society of Tropical Medicine and Hygiene* **87**: 436–443.

Slutsker L, Taylor TE, Wirima JJ & Stekettee RW (1994) In-hospital morbidity and mortality due to malaria-associated severe anaemia in two areas of Malawi with different patterns of malaria infection. *Transactions of the Royal Society of Tropical Medicine & Hygiene* **88**: 548–551.

Smith T, Armstrong-Schellenberg JRM & Hayes RC (1994) Attributable fraction estimates and case definitions for malaria in endemic areas. *Statistical Medicine* **13**: 2345–2358.

Snounou G, Pinheiro L, Goncalves A et al (1993) The importance of sensitive detection of malaria parasites in the human and insect hosts in epidemiological studies, as shown by the analysis of field samples from Guinea Bissau. *Transactions of the Royal Society of Tropical Medicine and Hygiene* **87**: 649–653.

Snow RW, Armstrong JRM, Forster D et al (1992) Childhood deaths in Africa: uses and limitations of verbal autopsies. *Lancet* **340**: 351–356.

Snow RW, Bastos de Azevedo I, Lowe BS et al (1994) Severe childhood malaria in two areas of markedly different falciparum transmission in East Africa. *Acta Tropica* **57**: 289–300.

Spielman A & Perrone JB (1989) Rapid diagnosis of malaria. *Lancet* **i:** 727.

Stone WJ, Hanchett JE & Knepshield JN (1972) Acute renal insufficiency due to falciparum malaria. *Archives of Internal Medicine* **129:** 620–628.

Subramanian D, Moise KJ & White AC (1992) Imported malaria in pregnancy: report of four cases and review of management. *Clinical Infectious Diseases* **15:** 408–413.

Taylor TE, Molyneux ME, Wirima JJ et al (1988) Blood glucose levels in Malawian children before and during the administration of intravenous quinine for severe falciparum malaria. *New England Journal of Medicine* **319:** 1040–1047.

Taylor TE, Borgstein A & Molyneux ME (1993a) Acid-base status in paediatric *Plasmodium falciparum* malaria. *Quarterly Journal of Medicine* **86:** 99–109.

Taylor TE, Wills BA, Kazembe P et al (1993b) Rapid coma resolution with artemether in Malawian children with cerebral malaria. *Lancet* **341:** 661–662.

Trang TTM, Nguyen HP, Ha V et al (1992) Acute renal failure in patients with severe falciparum malaria. *Clinical Infectious Diseases* **15:** 874–880.

Treutiger C-J, Hedlund I, Helmby H et al (1992) Rosette formation in *Plasmodium falciparum* isolates and anti-rosette activity of sera from Gambians with cerebral or uncomplicated malaria. *American Journal of Tropical Medicine and Hygiene* **46(5):** 503–510.

Waller D, Crawley J, Nosten F et al (1991) Intracranial pressure in childhood cerebral malaria. *Transactions of the Royal Society of Tropical Medicine and Hygiene* **85:** 362–364.

Warrell DA (1993) Clinical features of malaria. In Gilles HM & Warrell DA (eds) *Bruche-Chwatt's Essential Malariology*, 3rd edn, pp 35–49. London: Edward Arnold.

Warrell DA, Looareesuwan S, Warrell MJ et al (1982) Dexamethasone proves deleterious in cerebral malaria: a double blind trial in 100 comatose patients. *New England Journal of Medicine* **306:** 313–319.

Wernsdorfer WH & McGregor I (eds) (1988) *Malaria: Principles and Practice of Malariology.* Edinburgh: Churchill Livingstone.

White NJ (1986) Pathophysiology. In Strickland GT (ed.) *Clinics in Tropical Medicine and Communicable Diseases: Malaria*, pp 55–90. London: WB Saunders.

White NJ (1991) Lumbar puncture in cerebral malaria. *Lancet* **338:** 640–641 (letter).

White NJ, Warrell DA, Chanthavanich P et al (1983) Severe hypoglycemia and hyperinsulinemia in falciparum malaria. *New England Journal of Medicine* **309:** 61–66.

White NJ, Miller KD, Marsh K et al (1987) Hypoglycaemia in African children with severe malaria. *Lancet* **329:** 708–711.

White NJ, Looareesuwan S, Phillips RE et al (1988) Single dose phenobarbitone prevents convulsions in cerebral malaria. *Lancet* **332:** 64–66.

Whittle HC, Brown J, Marsh K et al (1984) T-cell control of Epstein–Barr virus infected B cells is lost during *P. falciparum* malaria. *Nature* **312:** 449–450.

Wilairatana P, Looareesuwan S, Vanijanonta S et al (1994) Hepatic metabolism in severe falciparum malaria: caffeine clearance study. *Annals of Tropical Medicine and Parasitology* **88(1):** 13–19.

Wirima JJ & Harries AD (1987) Absence of fever in non-immune patients developing falciparum malaria. *British Medical Journal* **295:** 913.

Wongrichanalai C, Chuanak N, Webster HK & Timasarn K (1992) Rapid test for malaria diagnosis. *Lancet* **i:** 1176.

World Health Organization (1990) Severe and complicated malaria. *Transactions of the Royal Society of Tropical Medicine and Hygiene* **84 (supplement 2):** 1–65.

World Health Organization (1991) *Basic Malaria Microscopy.* Geneva: World Health Organization.

World Health Organization (1993) *A Global Strategy for Malaria Control.* Geneva: World Health Organization.

Yorke W & Macfie J (1924) Observations on malaria made during treatment of general paralysis. *Transactions of the Royal Society of Tropical Medicine and Hygiene* **18:** 13–33.

5

Anti-malarial chemotherapy

PETER A. WINSTANLEY

Malaria remains as much a scourge as ever, primarily to the estimated 2 000 000 000 people who live in endemic areas, but also to travellers. Of the four species of Plasmodia capable of infecting man it is *Plasmodium falciparum* with which we have most problems: this species not only causes life-threatening illness but has also developed resistance to most classes of anti-malarial drugs. Consequently, the bulk of this chapter is devoted to the treatment of falciparum malaria.

TREATMENT OF CEREBRAL MALARIA

Principles of management

Established cerebral malaria is a medical emergency with about 10% mortality even in centres of excellence (Warrell et al, 1990): the chances of surviving without brain damage are optimized by appropriate use of anti-malarial drugs (quinine, quinidine and artemisinin derivatives; resistance to chloroquine is widespread and alternatives should be used if possible) and careful supportive treatment.

Quinine

Quinine (which is uneconomic to synthesize, and is therefore still extracted from Cinchona bark) is the drug of choice for severe malaria at present, mainly because of the low risk of encountering quinine-resistant organisms, rather than because of its potency; the 50% inhibitory concentration (IC50) of quinine against chloroquine-sensitive *P. falciparum* isolates is generally higher than for chloroquine. Unfortunately, sensitivity to quinine in parts of Indochina is declining (White, 1992) and treatment failures can probably be anticipated in this region in coming years.

The mode of action of quinine is unclear. Its effects are largely confined to sequestered trophozoites and, while its pharmacological action is less restricted than that of pyrimethamine/sulphadoxine (PM/SD; Fansidar™), it has little action on rings either in vitro (ter Kuile et al, 1993a) or ex vivo (Watkins et al, 1991); the decline of parasitaemia during the early phase of treatment seems to reflect sequestration of live parasites rather than killing.

Baillière's Clinical Infectious Diseases—
Vol. 2, No. 2, July 1995
ISBN 0–7020–1983–6

Quinine's clinical effects are often said to be rapid in onset, but the rate of parasite clearance achieved by quinine is lower than that of chloroquine (White et al, 1989) or artemisinin derivatives (White and Krishna, 1990), and similar to that of PM/SD (Winstanley et al, 1992). A rise in parasitaemia in the first 24 hours of treatment is common, does not necessarily indicate treatment failure, and is not an indication to change drug. However, after 24 hours, asexual parasitaemia should decline rapidly, clearing within 5 days. Gametocytes may persist thereafter, but they are not pathogenic and their presence does not imply treatment failure.

Most work on the pharmacokinetics of quinine in adults has been done in Thailand, and most work in children has been carried out in Africa. The effect of racial group on quinine disposition is not suspected to be large. However, parasite sensitivity to quinine varies geographically (the least sensitive parasites being found in parts of Indochina) and dose recommendations often reflect this. For cerebral malaria presenting in Europe and North America, regimens A and B in Table 1 are currently standard. When

Table 1. Quinine dose regimens studied in patients with cerebral malaria.

i.v. administration to Thai adults[a,b]

(A) 7 mg/kg i.v. by infusion pump over 30 minutes, followed immediately by 10 mg/kg (diluted in crystalloid) by infusion over 4 hours. Then 10 mg/kg infusions repeated 8 hourly to complete treatment[c], or until oral administration becomes possible.

(B) 20 mg/kg i.v. by infusion over 4 hours, followed by 10 mg/kg over 2 hours. Then 10 mg/kg infusions repeated 8 hourly to complete treatment[c], or until oral administration becomes possible.

i.v. administration to African children[d,e]

(C) 7.5 mg/kg by infusion pump over 30 minutes, followed immediately by 7.5 mg/kg (diluted in crystalloid) by infusion over 1.5 hours. Thereafter 10 mg/kg, infused over 2 hours, and repeated 12 hourly to complete treatment[c], or until oral anti-malarial drugs become possible.

(D) 15 mg/kg (diluted in crystalloid) by infusion over 2 hours. Thereafter, 10 mg/kg infused over 2 hours, and repeated 12 hourly to complete treatment[c], or until oral anti-malarial drugs become possible.

i.m. administration to Thai adults[f]

(E) 20 mg/kg by deep injection (2 sites) into the anterior thighs, and 8 hourly thereafter by 10 mg/kg injections (1 site) continued to complete treatment[c], or until oral drugs become possible.

i.m. administration to African children[d]

(F) 15 mg/kg by deep injection (2 sites) into the anterior thighs, and 12 hourly thereafter by 10 mg/kg injections (1 site) continued to complete treatment[c], or until oral drugs become possible.

Doses are expressed as mg of quinine dihydrochloride per kg body weight.
For administration to Thai adults either regimen (A) or regimen (B) should be chosen.
For administration to African children either regimen (C) or regimen (D) should be chosen.
[a] Davis et al, (1988).
[b] White et al (1983b).
[c] Seven day courses are usual in Indochina, where drug sensitivity may be falling. In Africa, 5 day courses seem adequate, but it is often more convenient to complete oral therapy with a long-acting drug such as pyrimethamine/sulphadoxine.
[d] Winstanley et al (1993).
[e] Winstanley et al (1994).
[f] Waller et al (1990).

delivered intravenously (i.v.), quinine is initially confined to a small central compartment so there is the potential to achieve dangerously high plasma concentrations if the rate of delivery is too fast; quinine *must* be diluted and infused at a slow, constant rate (preferably 2 to 4 hours). The volume of distribution is smaller in children with cerebral malaria than in adults (Winstanley et al, 1993) and dose recommendations differ slightly (see Table 2). Quinine undergoes extensive hepatic biotransformation, less than 20% of the drug is excreted unchanged, and is eliminated with a half-time of about 11 hours in healthy subjects, 16 hours in patients with uncomplicated malaria and about 18 hours in those with cerebral malaria. Liver disease can reduce quinine clearance (Karbwang et al, 1993), but this should not cause doses to be reduced, the risk from cerebral malaria outweighs that from possible drug toxicity (Warrell et al, 1990).

If it proves impossible to supervise i.v. infusions adequately, quinine may be given intramuscularly (i.m.) (Schapira et al, 1993); scrupulous skin disinfection and use of sterile equipment are essential to prevent sepsis (Yen et al, 1994). Absorption half-time ($t_{1/2,\ abs}$) seems to vary with the drug concentration in the bolus; when diluted (1:5, v/v, in water) $t_{1/2,\ abs}$ is about 9 minutes (Winstanley et al, 1993) compared with about 37 minutes when undiluted (Waller et al, 1990). The effect of shock on the absorption of i.m. quinine has been incompletely studied.

Quinine is extensively bound to plasma protein, principally to α_1-acid-glycoprotein (AGP) (Silamut et al, 1985, 1991; Mansor et al, 1990, 1991). In health about 80% of quinine is bound, but in malaria AGP concentrations rise and 90 to 95% of quinine becomes bound; this is relevant because it is the free fraction that results in both therapeutic and toxic effects. Using free quinine concentration as a means of comparison between in vitro chemosensitivity (of Kenyan isolates) and achieved concentration in malaria and following overdose, an approximate, therapeutic range of 0.2 to 2.0 mg l^{-1} of the free drug has been calculated. This range can only be taken to apply to parasites of equivalent chemosensitivity.

When given by recommended regimens, quinine is relatively safe. Hypersensitivity reactions are rare, they include: rashes, thrombocytopenia, leukopenia, disseminated intravascular coagulopathy, haemolytic-uraemic syndrome, fever, bronchospasm and pancytopenia (see Pirmohamed and Winstanley, 1993). Concentration-dependent toxicity may be seen if dose recommendations are exceeded or if unmonitored infusions run too fast. Retinal toxicity is common after deliberate quinine overdose, but appears to be unusual when the drug is used for malaria. Like quinidine, but less potent, quinine is a Vaughan–Williams Class Ia antiarrhythmic agent, and depresses the pacemaker rate, conduction rate and excitability, and lengthens both the action potential and refractory period. Electrocardiographic (ECG) features of toxicity include prolongation of the *QT* interval, widening of QRS complexes and non-specific T wave changes. Serious cardiovascular compromise is unusual except at very high drug concentrations, but may include: tachyarrhythmias, bradyarrhythmias and shock. At very high levels quinine can cause seizures. Both quinine and quinidine potentiate digoxin, flecainide and warfarin.

Quinidine

In the United States quinine is no longer available and cerebral malaria is treated with its diastereoisomer quinidine, which is readily available in American hospitals. Quinidine may be more potent against *P. falciparum* than quinine (Sabchareon et al, 1988), possibly because quinidine is less extensively bound to plasma protein than is quinine (Mihaly et al, 1987), and is certainly more cardiotoxic (White et al, 1983c); smaller doses are therefore recommended. Two regimens are available (Phillips et al, 1985; Miller et al, 1989). These are either (A) quinidine gluconate, 10 mg of the base per kg body weight by i.v. infusion over 2 hours, followed by 0.02 mg/kg/min by infusion pump for 72 hours, or until the patient can swallow, then quinine tablets to complete treatment, or (B) quinidine gluconate, 15 mg of the base per kg body weight by i.v. infusion over 4 hours, followed 8 hourly thereafter by 7.5 mg/kg until the patient can swallow, then quinine tablets to complete treatment.

Chloroquine

Chloroquine is a synthetic compound (easy to make and therefore very cheap) and remains the most widely used anti-malarial drug in the world, mainly for uncomplicated disease. Chloroquine's major drawback in life-threatening disease is drug-resistance and, where available, alternative drugs are strongly recommended. Against sensitive parasites, chloroquine is more potent than quinine (White et al, 1989), usually requires fewer doses to clear parasitaemia, does so faster and is better tolerated.

Chloroquine may act by inhibiting a putative plasmodial enzyme, haem polymerase (Slater and Cerami, 1992) which is responsible for polymerizing the toxic haem moiety ferriprotoporphyrin IX to form inert haemozoin. The mechanism by which *P. falciparum* develops resistance to chloroquine does not seem to concern the target enzyme; resistant parasites accumulate less chloroquine than sensitive parasites, although whether the mechanism involves faster expulsion of the drug (Krogstad et al, 1987) or slower entry (Bray et al, 1992) is contentious. The demonstration that some drugs, notably calcium channel antagonists and anti-histamines, can 'reverse' resistance to chloroquine in vitro has not yet been translated into clinical benefit, but work in this area continues.

In cerebral malaria cases, chloroquine may be given i.v. (as a slow constant-rate infusion), i.m., subcutaneously (s.c.) or, if parenteral use is impossible, via a nasogastric tube (White et al, 1988). The disposition of chloroquine is complicated. When delivered i.v. the drug is first distributed into a small central compartment (this probably has no anatomical correlate), so that there is the potential to achieve dangerously high plasma concentrations if delivery is too fast. Thereafter, chloroquine is distributed into progressively larger compartments, and is eliminated very slowly (its half-life from ranges 30 to 60 days), mainly in the urine (as the unchanged drug and as pharmacologically-active metabolites). Although chloroquine is mainly cleared by the kidney, dose reduction is not recommended in patients with cerebral malaria and renal failure because distribution, rather than elimination, is the main determinant of drug levels. Table 2 lists various regimens for chloroquine treatment of cerebral malaria.

Table 2. Chloroquine dose regimens in cerebral malaria.

Intravenous regimen 1: 10 mg/kg (diluted in crystalloid) *constant-rate infusion* over 8 hours *followed immediately by* 15 mg/kg (diluted in crystalloid) *constant-rate infusion* over 24 hours
Intravenous regimen 2: 5 mg/kg (diluted in crystalloid) *constant-rate infusion* over 4 hours repeated every 12 hours to a total dose of 25 mg/kg (i.e. 5 doses)
Intramuscular/subcutaneous regimen: 3.5 mg/kg repeated every 6 hours to a total dose of 25 mg/kg (i.e. 7 doses)
Nasogastric regimen: 10 mg/kg followed by 5 mg/kg at an interval of 6, 24 and 48 hours after first administration.

Doses are expressed as mg of chloroquine base per kg body weight.

Chloroquine is absorbed rapidly i.m. and s.c. with t_{max} being between 20 and 90 minutes; the disposition of i.m./s.c. chloroquine has been incompletely studied in shocked patients. Nasogastric administration of chloroquine should not be used as a first choice (there may be gastric stasis) unless parenteral administration is impossible. In young Gambian children with severe malaria, many of whom had cerebral malaria, nasogastric chloroquine had a $t_{1/2,\ abs}$ of about 40 minutes, and median t_{max} was 7.5 hours.

The therapeutic range of chloroquine can only be estimated crudely. The minimal therapeutic plasma concentration for chloroquine-sensitive *P. falciparum* is probably about 30 µg/l. Toxicity may be manifest with concentrations greater than 1 mg/l and after deliberate self-poisoning survival is rare with concentrations higher than 8 mg/l (Riou et al, 1988). There is evidence that the rate of rise of concentration is also an important determinant of symptomatic toxicity.

Chloroquine is usually well-tolerated when dose recommendations are followed. Rapid i.v. administration causes life-threatening cardiovascular toxicity which may include: cardiorespiratory arrest, hypotension (caused by reduced stroke volume and vasodilatation), tachyarrhythmias, bradyarrhythmias and ECG complex abnormalities. Neurological effects, observable in the already unconscious patient, include seizures and cerebral oedema. Other effects of toxicity discernable in the comatose patient include hypokalaemia, methaemoglobinaemia, and haemolysis in patients with glucose-6 phosphate dehydrogenase (G6PD)-deficiency.

Artemisinin and derivatives

Artemisinin (see White, 1994) is a pharmacologically-active molecule discovered in a herbal anti-malarial remedy. The drug itself remains in use, but several semi-synthetic derivatives have been developed, with the advantages of greater anti-malarial potency and stability, but the disadvantage of greater cost. Two of these, artemether and artesunate, have been available in China and Indochina for years and artemether is becoming widely available in Africa. None is yet licensed in Europe or the USA. Definitive recommendations on the optimal drug for cerebral malaria, its dose size, dose frequency and duration of treatment cannot yet be given; Table 3 summarizes some regimens which have been used for severe malaria.

Table 3. Some of the dose regimens of artemisinin, and derivatives, which have been used in cerebral malaria.

Drug	Route	Dose	Frequency and duration of treatment	Subsequent treatment
Artemisinin: Adults[a]	Suppository	600 to 1200 mg then 400 mg	Loading dose at 4, 24 and 48 hours	Mefloquine
Artesunate: Adults[a]	i.v.	2 mg/kg then 1 mg/kg	Loading dose at 12 and 24 hours	Mefloquine
Artemether: Children[b]	i.m.	3.2 mg/kg then 1.6 mg/kg	Loading dose daily for 4 days	Fansidar™ if full 5 days artemether interrupted

[a] See White (1994) for individual studies.
[b] Regimen used in the WHO-supported multi-centre African study.

Artemisinin is cheap to produce, but about five times less potent than its derivatives. No parenteral formulation is available, but for cerebral malaria it has been used successfully in suppository form. Artemether, which is more expensive than the 'parent drug' is used in cerebral malaria as an i.m. injection. Artesunate, also more expensive than artemisinin, is available for i.v. and i.m. injection. Artesunate is unstable and is therefore dispensed as powdered artesunic acid, which is dissolved in sodium bicarbonate immediately before use; attention to detail in its preparation is essential if it is to go into solution properly. All three compounds seem to be metabolized to dihydroartemisinin, a pharmacologically-active metabolite. In parts of Indochina, where multiple-drug-resistant *P. falciparum* is common, artemisinin derivatives have an invaluable role for both severe and uncomplicated falciparum malaria. In other parts of the tropics, where quinine retains acceptable efficacy against the parasite, the role of artemisinin derivatives is less clear.

The mode of action of artemisinin and its derivatives is unknown, but it has been suggested that intraparasitic iron catalyses the cleavage of the peroxide bridge, common to artemisinin and all derivatives, generating free radicals which form covalent bonds with parasite proteins. Artemisinin derivatives seem to have activity earlier in the maturation of the parasite than quinine or chloroquine (ter Kuile et al, 1993a), and achieve more rapid rates of decline in parasite count, suggestive of in vivo effects on circulating ring-forms. This observation may be important because, although the circulating parasites cause little pathology, they probably remain available for sequestration if the patient is treated with 'conventional' drugs such as quinine. This parasitological advantage of artemisinin derivatives may be accompanied by clinical advantages, since they are associated with a mean shortening of the time to fever clearance. Whether the mortality rate of cerebral malaria treated with artemisinin derivatives is lower than with quinine is unknown, and we await a study powerful enough to detect a difference. One disadvantage of this drug group is high recrudescence rates if therapy is shorter than 5 days in duration; there is no generally accepted explanation for this.

Although drug analytical methods have been developed, the pharmacokinetics of artemisinin derivatives have been incompletely described. This is principally due to the instability of the compounds in biological fluids, particularly in the presence of iron-containing molecules such as ferriprotoporphyrin (Muhia et al, 1994). However, although the therapeutic index of the drug class is not known precisely it appears to be large, pharmacokinetic data are therefore less essential to avoid toxicity than is the case for quinine or chloroquine. Similarly, pharmacokinetic data are unlikely to help us increase further the rate of parasite clearance in patients given artemisinin derivatives, this seems pretty maximal already. In contrast, reliable pharmacokinetic data may help explain early recrudescence, and may help develop better dosing schedules.

Unlike chloroquine and quinine, dose-related toxicity seems to be unusual with artemisinin derivatives; fever is the only common problem. However, in dogs, high doses (20 mg/kg per day) of artemether and arteether given for prolonged periods (8 days) caused defects in the pons and medulla (Weshe et al, 1994). Whether such toxicity will be seen in man, particularly upon frequent repeat exposure, is unknown.

TREATMENT OF UNCOMPLICATED FALCIPARUM MALARIA

In many countries uncomplicated falciparum malaria is the commonest cause of hospital attendance. Unless properly treated malaria threatens the lives of young children, the fetuses of pregnant women and the income of bread-winners; it is thus of great importance to public health.

Chloroquine-sensitive parasites

In view of widespread resistance, chloroquine cannot be recommended for non-immune patients with uncomplicated falciparum malaria, including those cases imported into Europe and North America. However, in many malaria-endemic countries, chloroquine remains the drug of first choice. This continued use of chloroquine is the product of extremely difficult health care decisions on deployment of scarce resources—malaria is only one of many health care problems, and even PM/SD costs more than chloroquine.

The standard regimen is 10 mg/kg (of the base), followed by 5 mg/kg after 6 hours and by 5 mg/kg on the second and third days of treatment. This regimen is usually well-tolerated, although it can be difficult to persuade children to take the very bitter syrup. Symptomatic adverse effects include gastrointestinal upset, blurring of vision (usually due to changes in refraction—corneal accumulation of chloroquine is often asymptomatic), dizziness and rash. Pruritus, although uncommon in whites, is very common in blacks and may cause poor compliance. There is no evidence that pruritus is dose-related and it is usually unaccompanied by rash. None of these reactions is usually severe enough to warrant cessation of treatment, especially if no alternative drugs are available. Chloroquine can cause retinopathy, but this is unusual if the total dose is less than 100 g, and in practice this is not achieved even by patients on long-term chemoprophylaxis.

Chloroquine-resistant parasites: pyrimethamine/sulphadoxine (Fansidar™)

PM/SD is used for uncomplicated malaria which has not been cured by chloroquine, or as first-line treatment where chloroquine has been dropped from use. PM/SD is cheap, practicable (only one dose is needed) and highly effective in much of Africa and South America. In much of Indochina, where parasites are often resistant to both PM and SD, PM/SD is clinically useless; resistance to PM has been reported in Africa (Landgraf et al, 1994) but resistance to both PM and SD seems to be unusual at the moment.

PM is a competitive inhibitor of dihydrofolate reductase (DHFR), the enzyme that reduces dihydrofolate to tetrahydrofolate. The amino acid sequence of DHFR differs between species, so that PM is considerably more potent against *P. falciparum* than mammalian cells. Unfortunately *P. falciparum* is capable of undergoing point mutations of the gene for DHFR, thereby becoming PM-resistant (Hyde, 1990). Like other sulphonamides, SD inhibits the incorporation of para-aminobenzoic acid (PABA) into dihydropteroate, a precursor of dihydrofolate, by competitive inhibition of dihydropteroate synthetase (DHPS). The amino acid sequence of plasmodial DHPS is currently the subject of active research; it is possible that resistance to SD is caused by point mutations of the gene for DHPS (Brooks et al, 1994), but work is at an early stage. In combination, PM and SD are synergistic.

In vitro and ex vivo, the effects of PM/SD are confined to late trophozoites. As a result, PM/SD is said to have a slow onset of action, and is not generally recommended for severe malaria, but the rate of parasite clearance achieved by PM/SD is about the same as that of quinine. Sensitive falciparum malaria is generally treated with a single oral dose of PM/SD (Table 4), which makes the treatment of out-patients very practicable. An i.m. formulation is available, and is used for patients with protracted vomiting; its efficacy in severe forms of childhood malaria has been compared favourably with that of quinine (Simao et al, 1991).

Table 4. Drugs for clinically uncomplicated, but drug-resistant falciparum malaria.

Drug	Areas where resistance to this drug is encountered	Regimen
Fansidar™ (Pyrimethamine + Sulphadoxine)	Indochina[a] Africa[b] South America[b]	Single dose Adults: 3 tablets[c] Children: pyrimethamine 1.25 mg/kg, sulphadoxine 25 mg/kg
Halofantrine	Indochina[b]	Adults[d]: 500 mg 6 hourly to a total dose of 1.5 g Children[e]: 8 mg/kg 6 hourly to a total dose of 24 mg/kg
Mefloquine	Indochina[b]	10 mg/kg (of the base) twice, 6 to 8 hours apart (total dose 20 mg/kg)

[a] The drug should not be used.
[b] Resistance is encountered, but the drug retains efficacy in a high proportion of cases.
[c] One tablet = pyrimethamine 25 mg, sulphadoxine 500 mg.
[d] 250 mg/tablet.
[e] Paediatric suspension 2 mg/ml (each dose is therefore 0.5 ml/kg).

Oral PM and SD are extensively and rapidly absorbed, with t_{max} being about 12 and 4 hours, respectively (Winstanley et al, 1992). PM, but not SD, is absorbed more slowly after i.m. injection, possibly because of its poor aqueous solubility. The elimination half-time of PM varies from 40 to 100 hours, and that of SD is about 200 hours. It is because of this slow elimination rate that PM/SD need only be given once.

In vitro concentration versus effect curves of PM and SD against *P. falciparum* are log-normal (although those of SD are highly dependent upon the concentrations of PABA and folic acid in the medium), but no relationship has been demonstrated between concentrations in vivo and clinical effect. Furthermore, the two are almost invariably used in synergistic combination, making such clinical assessment difficult. Consequently, there is no accepted therapeutic range.

PM has a large therapeutic index, but does cause toxicity in overdose. In children, fatalities have been reported with doses exceeding 375 mg (15 tablets of pyrimethamine/dapsone (Daraprim™) or pyrimethamine/sulphadoxine (Fansidar™)). Poisoning has been reported to cause coma, seizures, apnoea, pyrexia, visual impairment and deafness. Because PM causes concentration-dependent suppression of the marrow, temporary pancytopenia or agranulocytosis, can be anticipated in some patients. Treatment is confined to supportive care since there are no means of enhancing drug elimination. Patients should probably be given folinic acid. In contrast the effects of SD overdose are relatively mild, though methaemoglobinaemia can occur.

Hypersensitivity to PM is rare, but is common with sulphonamides and constitutes an absolute contraindication to the use of PM/SD. PM is teratogenic in animals, and teratogenicity has been reported in humans but the risk seems to be low. It is generally recommended that PM be avoided during the first trimester. Prophylactic PM/SD can cause severe skin reactions (including severe erythema multiforme and toxic epidermal necrolysis) and is no longer recommended. There are few data on the incidence rate of severe idiosyncratic adverse reactions to PM/SD when used for malaria treatment.

Multiple-drug-resistant parasites

Mefloquine

This synthetic drug has structural similarities to quinine. It is effective against *P. falciparum* strains resistant to chloroquine and PM/SD, and is therefore extensively used in Indochina. Unfortunately resistance to mefloquine is becoming common in parts of this region (Nosten et al, 1991; ter Kuile et al, 1992). Although it is marketed in some African countries, and is very potent against local *P. falciparum* strains, mefloquine is too expensive for widespread use. Its mode of action is unknown.

Mefloquine is formulated for oral use only. It is well absorbed even when given by nasogastric tube to patients with severe malaria (Chanthavanich et al, 1985) and t_{max} is under 12 hours. The drug is widely distributed and is extensively bound to plasma proteins. Mefloquine is eliminated, as the unchanged drug and as inactive metabolites, both in the urine and the bile; the elimination half-life is very long, being between 15 and 33 days. There is no established therapeutic range.

Because of the structural similarity between mefloquine and quinine, some authorities recommend that mefloquine should be withheld for 24 hours after quinine, and quinine loading doses are usually not given if mefloquine has been taken in the preceding few days. The exact risk of teratogenesis with mefloquine is unknown, but currently the drug is contraindicated for chemoprophylaxis in the first trimester of pregnancy, and the British National Formulary recommends that pregnancy should be avoided for 3 months after use. Mefloquine prophylaxis has been used in Indochina for pregnant women (over 20 weeks gestation). The risk of malaria was significantly reduced, and there was no increase in the risk of adverse outcome to the fetus (Nosten et al, 1994).

Features of mefloquine overdose have not been documented fully, but include vertigo, visual disturbance, hypotension and tachycardia. There are no accepted means of enhancing elimination, and the management of poisoning is mainly supportive. In standard chemotherapeutic doses, mefloquine can cause acute psychosis and seizures (especially in patients with previous seizures), but the prevalence rate is contentious; estimates range from 1 in 215 (Weinke et al, 1991) to 1 in 1754 (Luxemburger et al, 1991). The risk of neuropsychiatric events during mefloquine chemo-prophylaxis may be no higher than with chloroquine. Allergy to mefloquine is uncommon but rashes, some of them serious, have been reported.

Halofantrine

Halofantrine is effective against many strains of *P. falciparum* resistant to chloroquine, PM/SD and mefloquine, and is used extensively in parts of Indochina. It is rarely used in Africa because of its high cost. Unfortunately the sensitivity of Thai isolates is already diminishing (Nosten et al, 1993). Halofantrine is available only in oral formulations, but the paediatric suspension has the advantage over many anti-malarials of a pleasant taste. The mode of action of halofantrine is unknown. In vitro it has effects against sequestered stages. Ex vivo halofantrine, unlike quinine or PM/SD, appears to affect circulating ring-forms (Watkins et al, 1991).

Halofantrine is poorly, and variably, absorbed from the gut, and this may result in very large inter-individual differences in achieved plasma concentration, and may occasionally be responsible for drug failure (Karbwang et al, 1991). Absorption is markedly enhanced if the drug is given with fatty food (Milton et al, 1989), but this is of relatively little clinical value since many patients are anorectic and nauseated. When given via nasogastric tube to patients with severe falciparum malaria (who also received i.v. quinine), halofantrine was undetectable in the plasma of some patients (Watkins et al, 1995). Halofantrine is eliminated almost entirely by hepatic metabolism to an equipotent desbutyl metabolite. The elimination half-time varies between 1 and 4 days.

The in vitro IC50 of halofantrine is variable, the 'cutoff' defining resistance being taken as $4\,\mu M$, but whether in vitro figures can be used as therapeutic 'targets' in vivo, is unclear. Furthermore, although the drug does produce apparently dose-related cardiotoxicity, the 'toxic threshold', is unknown, and consequently there is no reliable therapeutic range.

Until quite recently halofantrine was not suspected to cause serious toxicity, reactions had been limited to pruritus, gastrointestinal upset, mild elevation of transaminases and occasional reports of mouth ulcer. However, prolongation of the QT_c interval has been added to the list. This was first noted in the setting of emerging resistance on the Thai–Burmese border, where the standard regimen (three 8 mg/kg doses 6 hours apart) was increased (to nine 8 mg/kg doses over 3 days) to reduce recrudescence rates. The high-dose regimen was associated with one cardiac death, which prompted a prospective study of ECG changes, and halofantrine dose-related lengthening of the QT_c interval (by more than 25%) was observed (Nosten et al, 1993).

Halofantrine is an inappropriate choice for chemoprophylaxis, but is used for 'presumptive self-treatment' by patients isolated from medical help. It is recommended that cardiological assessment (including an ECG) be undertaken before the drug is used in this way. In patients with established multi-resistant falciparum malaria the risk/benefit ratio differs, and treatment choices may well be limited. In patients with pre-existing QT_c prolongation halofantrine could be avoided, but other anti-malarials may not be risk-free either.

Quinine combinations

Quinine is usually effective against *P. falciparum* of any geographical origin, but is unpleasant (it is very bitter, and usually causes severe cinchonism—nausea, vertigo, deafness and tinnitus—at therapeutic drug levels) and must be taken frequently; 600 mg (adult dose) should be given every 8 hours by mouth. Another disadvantage of quinine therapy is its long treatment course (7 days is recommended for imported malaria), but this can be reduced (to 5 days) by combining it with other drugs. Fansidar™, tetracycline (*not* in children under 8 years), mefloquine and halofantrine may all be used.

Artemisinin and derivatives

In parts of Indochina even mefloquine and halofantrine may fail to clear asexual parasitaemia, and artemisinin derivatives are increasingly used for uncomplicated disease. In some areas the impetus is economic rather than parasitologic. For example, parasites in Vietnam may retain sensitivity to mefloquine, but this drug is unaffordable whereas locally grown and formulated artemisinin is inexpensive. There is a high risk of recrudescence if artemisinin derivatives are used alone.

TREATMENT OF INFECTIONS WITH *P. VIVAX, OVALE* AND *MALARIAE*

Plasmodium vivax, ovale and *malariae* cause disease which differs from falciparum malaria in two main ways: life-threatening illness is rare and sensitivity to chloroquine is usual (although chloroquine-resistant *P. vivax* does occur in Papua New Guinea) (Murphy et al, 1992). In addition, unlike *P. falciparum* or *P. malariae*, *P. vivax* and *P. ovale* have 'dormant' hepatic stages which, if untreated, may cause late relapse.

Clinical cure

This term denotes clinical improvement and disappearance of asexual forms from the blood. Chloroquine is the drug of first choice (doses as cited above), but *P. vivax*, *P. malariae* and *P. ovale* infections all respond to quinine, quinidine, mefloquine and halofantrine as well. Clinical response to antifolate anti-malarials, such as Fansidar™, is less predictable.

Radical cure of *P. vivax* and *P. ovale*: use of primaquine

Hepatic hypnozoites of these two species, although asymptomatic (and not associated with perturbation of liver function tests), are treated to prevent relapse. Drugs used for clinical cure do not eradicate hypnozoites; primaquine is the only effective drug currently available. The mode of action of this synthetic 8-aminoquiniline is unknown. It is rapidly and extensively absorbed from the gut, but undergoes extensive first-pass metabolism to pharmacologically-active derivatives. Primaquine and its metabolites are excreted predominantly in the bile, and undergo enterohepatic circulation. The elimination half-time is about 6 hours.

The usual adult regimen of primaquine is 15 mg daily for 14 days, started after clinical cure. Toxicity is frequent with doses greater than 60 mg (or 8 tablets of the phosphate salt) in one day, and include headache, nausea and abdominal pain.

Methaemoglobinaemia is common (particularly in G6PD-deficiency) and although usually mild, may cause severe compromise including cyanosis, tachypnoea and shock. Haemolytic anaemia, intravascular haemolysis and leukopenia may all occur, the first two especially in patients with G6PD-deficiency. Patients should be screened for G6PD status before treatment, and primaquine withheld from deficient patients; malaria relapses are probably safer than intravascular haemolysis.

FUTURE POSSIBILITIES

Priorities for anti-malarial drugs depend on your situation. In Africa, where most lives are lost, the need is for a cheap, effective and safe alternative to Fansidar™, whose redundancy cannot be far off. In Indochina, where multi-resistant *P. falciparum* is a major problem, the need is for reliable chemotherapy, and cost is less of an issue. The industrialized nations, which have the means to develop new drugs, need safe chemoprophylaxis for travellers and soldiers.

Atovaquone

This drug is not yet generally available, but is currently being studied in combination with proguanil (with which it synergizes) against multi-resistant falciparum malaria in Indochina. Atovaquone is given orally, but absorption is incomplete at high dosage. Clinical experience with the drug is still in its early stages, but it seems to be well tolerated.

Pyronaridine

This was developed in the 1970s in China and his drug is effective against some strains of multi-resistant *P. falciparum.*

Novel antifolate combinations

It seems likely that the useful lifetime of PM/SD in Africa will be short, but *P. falciparum* develops resistance to DHFR-inhibitors by relatively drug-specific, genetically-determined variation in the enzyme, and sensitivity to other DHFR-inhibitors may be retained. The potential of these drugs is currently being studied.

SUMMARY

This chapter covers the clinical use of antimalarial drugs for severe and uncomplicated falciparum malaria, and for malaria due to *P. vivax, ovale* and *malariae.*

Parenteral quinine is the drug of first choice for severe falciparum malaria. If given intravenously, quinine must be diluted and given by slow infusion; quinine may also be given intramuscularly. In parts of South East Asia, where sensitivity to quinine is declining, intramuscular artemether (or other artemisinin-derivatives) may become the drug of first-choice in the near future.

Uncomplicated falciparum malaria is most commonly treated with oral chloroquine but, because of widespread resistance, alternatives should be used if available. *Plasmodium falciparum* usually retains sensitivity to pyrimethamine/sulphadoxine (Fansidar™) in Africa, but is usually resistant in South East Asia, where quinine, mefloquine or halofantrine are usually required.

Plasmodium ovale and *malariae*, and most *P. vivax* are sensitive to chloroquine. To prevent recurrence (from dormant liver stages) patients with *P. vivax* or *ovale* infections are given primaquine, after checking their glucose-6-phosphate dehydrogenase status.

REFERENCES

Bray PG, Howells RE & Ward SA (1992) Vacuolar acidification and chloroquine sensitivity in *Plasmodium falciparum*. *Biochemical Pharmacology* **43**: 1219–1227.

Brooks DR, Wang P, Read M et al (1994) Sequence variation of the hydroxymethyldihydropterin pyrophosphokinase: dihydropteroate synthetase gene in lines of the human malaria parasite *Plasmodium falciparum*, with differing resistance to sulfadoxine. *European Journal of Biochemistry* **224**: 397–405.

Chanthavanich P, Looareesuwan S, White NJ et al (1985) Intragastric mefloquine is absorbed rapidly in patients with cerebral malaria. *American Journal of Tropical Medicine* **34**: 1028–1036.

Davis TME, White NJ, Looareesuwan S & et al (1988) Quinine pharmacokinetics in cerebral malaria: predicted plasma concentrations after rapid intravenous loading using a two-compartment model. *Transactions of the Royal Society of Tropical Medicine and Hygiene* **82**: 542–547.

Hyde JE (1990) The dihydrofolate-thymidylate synthetase gene in the drug resistance of malaria parasites. *Pharmacology and Therapeutics* **48**: 45–59.

Karbwang J, Milton KA, Na-Bangchang K et al (1991) Pharmacokinetics of halofantrine in Thai patients with acute uncomplicated falciparum malaria. *British Journal of Clinical Pharmacology* **31**: 484–487.

Karbwang J, Thanavibul A, Molunto P & Na-Bangchang K (1993) The pharmacokinetics of quinine in patients with hepatitis. *British Journal of Clinical Pharmacology* **35**: 444–446.

Krishna S, Ter Kuile F, Supanaranond W et al (1993) Pharmacokinetics, efficacy and toxicity of parenteral halofantrine in uncomplicated malaria. *British Journal of Clinical Pharmacology* **36**: 585–591.

Krogstad DJ, Gluzman I, Kyle D et al (1987) Efflux of chloroquine from *Plasmodium falciparum*: mechanism of chloroquine resistance. *Science* **235**: 1283–1285.

Landgraf B, Kollaritsch H, Wiedermann G & Wernsdorfer WH (1994) *Plasmodium falciparum*: susceptibility *in-vitro* and *in-vivo* to chloroquine and sulfadoxine-pyrimethamine in Ghanaian schoolchildren. *Transactions of the Royal Society of Tropical Medicine and Hygiene* **88**: 440–442.

Luxemberger C, Nosten F, Ter Kuile F et al (1991) Mefloquine for multi-drug-resistant malaria. *Lancet* **338**: 1268.

Mansor SM, Taylor TE, McGrath CS et al 1990. The safety and kinetics of intramuscular quinine in Malawian children with moderately severe falciparum malaria. *Transactions of the Royal Society of Tropical Medicine and Hygiene* **84**: 482–488.

Mansor SM, Molyneux ME, Taylor TE et al (1991) Effect of *Plasmodium falciparum* malaria infection on the plasma concentration of alpha$_1$ acid glycoprotein and the binding of quinine in Malawian children. *British Journal of Clinical Pharmacology* 32: 317–323.

Mihaly GW, Ching MS, Klejn M et al (1987) Differences in the binding of quinine and quinidine to plasma proteins. *British Journal of Clinical Pharmacology* 24: 769–774.

Miller KD, Greenberg A & Campbell CC (1989) Treatment of severe malaria in the United States with a continuous infusion of quinidine gluconate and exchange transfusion. *New England Journal of Medicine* 321: 65–70.

Milton KA, Edwards G, Ward SA et al (1989) Pharmacokinetics of halofantrine in man: effects of food and dose size. *British Journal of Clinical Pharmacology* 28: 71–77.

Molyneux ME, Taylor TE, Wirima JJ & Borgstein J (1989) Clinical features and prognostic indicators in paediatric cerebral malaria: a study of 131 comatose Malawian children. *Quarterly Journal of Medicine* 71: 441–459.

Muhia DK, Thomas CG, Ward SA et al (1994) Ferriprotoporphyrin catalysed decomposition of artemether: analytical and pharmacological implications. *Biochemical Pharmacology* 48: 889–895.

Murphy GS, Basri H, Purnomo A et al (1992) Vivax malaria resistant to treatment and prophylaxis with chloroquine. *Lancet* 341: 96–100.

Nosten F, Ter Kuile F, Chongsuphajaisiddhi T et al (1991) Mefloquine-resistant falciparum malaria on the Thai/Burmese border. *Lancet* 337: 1140–1143.

Nosten F, Ter Kuile F, Luxemburger C et al (1993) Cardiac effects of antimalarial treatment with halofantrine. *Lancet* 341: 1054–1056.

Nosten F, Ter Kuile F, Maelankiri L et al (1994) Mefloquine prophylaxis prevents malaria during pregnancy: a double-blind, placebo-controlled study. *Journal of Infectious Diseases* 169: 595–603.

Pasvol G, Newton CRJC, Winstanley PA et al (1992) Quinine treatment of severe falciparum malaria in African children; a randomised trial of three regimens. *American Journal of Tropical Medicine and Hygiene* 45: 702–713.

Phillips RE, Warrell DA, White NJ et al (1985) Intravenous quinidine for the treatment of severe falciparum malaria. *New England Journal of Medicine* 1985; 312: 1273–1278.

Pirmohamed M & Winstanley PA (1993) Antiprotozoal drugs. In Aronson JK & van Boxtel CJ, (eds) *Meyler's Side Effects of Drugs Annual* 1993, pp 325–336. Amsterdam: Elsevier.

Riou B, Barriot P, Rimailho A & Baud F. (1988) Treatment of severe chloroquine poisoning. *New England Journal of Medicine* 318: 1–6.

Sabchareon A, Chongsuphajaisiddhi T & Attanath P (1982) Serum quinine concentrations following the initial dose in children with falciparum malaria. *Southeast Asian Journal of Tropical Medicine and Public Health* 13: 556–562.

Schapira A, Solomon T, Julien M et al (1993) Comparison of intramuscular and intravenous quinine for the treatment of severe and complicated malaria in children. *Transactions of the Royal Society of Tropical Medicine and Hygiene* 87: 299–302.

Silamut K, White NJ, Looareesuwan S & Warrell DA (1985) Binding of quinine to plasma proteins in falciparum malaria. *American Journal of Tropical Medicine and Hygiene* 34: 681–686.

Silamut K, Molunto P, Ho M et al (1991) Alpha$_1$ acid glycoprotein [orosomucoid] and plasma protein binding of quinine in falciparum malaria. *British Journal of Clinical Pharmacology* 32: 311–317.

Simao F, Macome A, Pateguana F & Schapira A (1991) Comparison of intramuscular sulfadoxine-pyrimethamine and intramuscular quinine for the treatment of falciparum malaria in children. *Transactions of the Royal Society of Tropical Medicine and Hygiene* 85: 341–344.

Slater AF & Cerami A (1992) Inhibition by chloroquine of a novel haem polymerase enzyme activity in malaria trophozoites. *Nature* 355: 108–109.

ter Kuile F, Nosten F, Thieren M et al (1992) High-dose mefloquine in the treatment of multi-drug-resistant falciparum malaria. *Journal of Infectious Diseases* 166: 1393–1400.

ter Kuile F, White NJ, Holloway P et al (1993a) In-vitro pharmacodynamics of drugs used for the treatment of severe malaria. *Experimental Parasitology* 76: 85–95.

ter Kuile FO, Dolan G & Nosten F (1993b) Halofantrine versus mefloquine in treatment of multidrug-resistant falciparum malaria. *Lancet* i: 1044–1049.

Waller D, Krishna S, Craddock C et al (1990) The pharmacokinetic properties of intramuscular quinine in Gambian children with severe falciparum malaria. *Transactions of the Royal Society of Tropical Medicine and Hygiene* 84: 488–491.

Warrell DA, Molyneux ME, Beales PF et al (1990) Severe and complicated malaria. *Transactions of the Royal Society of Tropical Medicine and Hygiene*. **84: (supplement 2)**.

Watkins WM, Woodrow C & Marsh K (1991) Falciparum malaria: differential effects of antimalarial drugs on ex vivo parasite viability during the critical early phase of therapy. *American Journal of Tropical Medicine and Hygiene* **49:** 106–12

Watkins WM, Winstanley PA, Murphy SA et al (1995) Halofantrine pharmacokinetics in Kenyan children with complicated and uncomplicated falciparum malaria. *British Journal of Clinical Pharmacology* **39:** 283–289.

Weshe DL, DeCoster MA, Tortella FC & Brewer TG (1994) Neurotoxicity of artemisinin analogs *in vitro*. *Antimicrobial Agents and Chemotherapy* **38:** 1813–1819.

Weinke T, Trautmann M, Held T et al (1991) Neuropsychiatric side effects of mefloquine. *American Journal of Tropical Medicine and Hygiene* **45:** 86–91.

White NJ (1992) Antimalarial drug resistance: the pace quickens. *Journal of Antimicrobial Chemotherapy* **30:** 571–585.

White NJ (ed.) (1994) Artemisinin. *Transactions of the Royal Society of Tropical Medicine and Hygiene* **88: (supplement 1)**.

White NJ & Krishna S (1990) Treatment of malaria: some considerations and limitations of the current methods of assessment. *Transactions of the Royal Society of Tropical Medicine and Hygiene* **83:** 767–778.

White NJ, Looareesuwan S, Warrell DA et al (1982) Quinine pharmacokinetics and toxicity in cerebral and uncomplicated falciparum malaria. *American Journal of Medicine* **73:** 564–571.

White NJ, Chanthavanich P, Krishna S et al (1983a) Quinine disposition kinetics. *British Journal of Clinical Pharmacology* **16:** 399–404.

White NJ, Looareesuwan S, Warrell DA et al (1983b) Quinine loading dose in cerebral malaria. *American Journal of Tropical Medicine and Hygiene* **32:** 1–5.

White NJ, Looareesuwan S & Warrell DA (1983c) Quinine and quinidine: a comparison of ECG effects during the treatment of malaria. *Journal of Cardiovascular Pharmacology* **5:** 173–175.

White NJ, Miller K, Churchill F et al (1988) Chloroquine treatment of severe malaria in children: pharmacokinetics, toxicity and new dosage recommendations. *New England Journal of Medicine* **319:** 1493–1500.

White NJ & Krishna S, Waller D et al (1989) Open comparison of intramuscular chloroquine and quinine in children with severe chloroquine-sensitive falciparum malaria. *Lancet* **ii:** 1313–1316.

Winstanley PA, Watkins WM, Newton CRJC et al (1992) The disposition of oral and intramuscular pyrimethamine-sulphadoxine in Kenyan children with high parasitaemia but clinically non-severe falciparum malaria. *British Journal of Clinical Pharmacology* **33:** 143–148.

Winstanley PA, Newton CR, Watkins WM et al (1993) Towards optimal parenteral quinine regimens for young children with cerebral malaria: importance of unbound quinine concentration. *Transactions of the Royal Society of Tropical Medicine and Hygiene* **87:** 201–206.

Winstanley PA, Mberu MK, Watkins WM et al (1994) Towards optimal regimens of parenteral quinine for young African children with cerebral malaria: unbound quinine concentrations following a simple loading dose regimen. *Transactions of the Royal Society of Tropical Medicine and Hygiene* **88:** 577–580.

Yen LM, Dao LM, Day NP et al (1994) Role of quinine in the high mortality of intramuscular injection tetanus. *Lancet* **344:** 786–787.

6

Controversies in the management of severe falciparum malaria

NICHOLAS J. WHITE

The management of severe falciparum malaria generates more than its fair share of controversy. Since the recognition, some 350 years ago, that the bark of the Cinchona tree from the Peruvian Andes could cure certain fevers, there has been disagreement about the optimum dose regimen for the Cinchona alkaloids, the incidence and severity of adverse effects and the additional treatments that were required for the severely ill patient. Until Meckel (1847) and Virchow (1849) associated haemozoin (malaria pigment) with periodic fever, and Laveran (1880) identified the intra-erythrocytic parasite as the cause of malaria, the alkaloids of the Cinchona bark were used empirically for the treatment of fever. Doses ranged from the homeopathic to the industrial, and opinion varied considerably on the risks and benefits of this treatment. With standardized horticultural practices, improved pharmaceutical processes, and the early development of clinical trials, dose regimens for quinine (the principal anti-malarial alkaloid) became standardized and a measure of consensus was achieved. However, controversy continued as to the optimum route of administration in severely ill patients. Oral administration was unreliable, the rectal route was irritant, subcutaneous injection caused skin necrosis, and rapid intra-venous injection was often followed by collapse. Ronald Ross, amongst many, considered that administration by intramuscular injection was dangerous and should not be used, largely because the dihydrochloride salt required for aqueous solution is acidic, and causes tissue necrosis (Ross, 1914; Fletcher and Visuvalingam, 1923). Intramuscular quinine was (and still is) an important cause of tetanus (Yen et al, 1994). 'Buffered' salts for intramuscular injection were then developed and these are still widely used today (particularly in Francophone Africa). Quinine was known to be hypotensive when given by intravenous injection, although this could be avoided by giving the drug slowly. The method of slow intravenous infusion of quinine proved safe and effective in the Japanese Prisoner-of-War camps and became the method of choice for the treatment of severe malaria in resistant areas (Strahan, 1948). After the second World War chloroquine gradually replaced quinine as the treatment of choice for all species of human malaria, and also for severe malaria, although quinine was still used extensively in Francophone Africa.

Baillière's Clinical Infectious Diseases—
Vol. 2, No. 2, July 1995
ISBN 0–7020–1983–6

309

The gradual spread of chloroquine resistance in the 1960s and 1970s necessitated a reversion from chloroquine to quinine as the treatment of choice for severe falciparum malaria. With increasing availability of blood concentration measurements of quinine (a relatively easy procedure because of the intrinsic fluorescence of the compound) it became apparent that patients with severe malaria had considerably higher blood concentrations than volunteers or patients with uncomplicated malaria. This resulted in a recommendation that doses should be reduced in patients with severe malaria (Hall, 1976, 1977). But, more detailed pharmacokinetic studies conducted in the 1980s (White et al, 1982) led to opposite conclusions and a revision of this recommendation, namely the introduction of the use of an initial loading dose in severe disease (White et al, 1983a). After chloroquine emerged as the treatment of choice for all malaria worldwide in the 1950s, there were very few studies of its pharmacokinetic or pharmacodynamic properties, and there was no information in severe malaria. However, the abrupt announcement by the World Health Organization in 1984 that parenteral chloroquine was 'no longer recommended in severe malaria because it was considered dangerous (WHO, 1984)', prompted a series of prospective studies of chloroquine pharmacology (Watt et al, 1987; White et al, 1987, 1988a). These also led to a clear definition of a therapeutic ratio, a reversal of the proscription, and a revision of the recommendations for the use of parenteral chloroquine so that the risks of iatrogenic hypotension could be minimized (WHO, 1986a, 1990; White et al, 1987, 1988a). In the 1990s we have seen the introduction of compounds from China related to artemisinin (Hien and White, 1993), and continued uncertainty and debate over the relative merits of the different anti-malarial drugs and the optimum dose regimens.

Over the past century many ancillary treatments have been suggested for severe falciparum malaria, but none has been shown unequivocally to improve outcome. Many of these adjunctive therapies have been suggested on the basis of incomplete or incorrect understanding of the pathophysiology of severe falciparum malaria (not that we fully understand it yet!), and also the considerable disparities between relatively rich temperate countries where a few non-immune adult expatriates return each year with severe falciparum malaria, and the vast majority of cases who are seen in the poor rural tropics against a background of repeated infections and partial immunity. As a result, anecdotal experiences based on small numbers of adult cases managed in modern intensive care units, are extrapolated to the tropics, where the majority of cases are in childhood, and facilities are, at best, limited. The use of high dose corticosteroids in the treatment of cerebral malaria was an example of this phenomenon.

STEROIDS IN CEREBRAL MALARIA

Cerebral oedema is a common finding at postmortem examination in fatal cases of cerebral malaria. The original suggestions of Rigdon (1944) that cerebral oedema might play a primary pathological role in cerebral malaria, were taken up by Maegraith and colleagues in Liverpool (Maegraith and Fletcher, 1972). This group conducted a series of studies in simian malaria (*Plasmodium knowlesi*) which showed that there was an increase in blood–brain barrier permeability in severe malaria that could be reversed by both steroids and chloroquine. However, the rhesus monkey (*Macaca mulatta*) with lethal *P. knowlesi* malaria does not develop an encephalopathy similar to cerebral malaria in man. (Indeed despite recent claims for the sequestering simian parasites *P. coatneyi* and *P. fragile* in rhesus monkeys, there is no good animal model of cerebral malaria that reproduces both the clinical and pathological features of the disease in man.) Furthermore chloroquine, which reversed the permeability abnormality in the monkey, was ineffective clinically against chloroquine-resistant strains of *P. falciparum* causing cerebral malaria. Nevertheless, after some preliminary experience in severe falciparum malaria in western intensive care units (Woodruff and Dickinson, 1968), high-dose corticosteroids were used increasingly throughout the world as adjunctive therapies in cerebral malaria. This practice stopped following a double-blind placebo-controlled evaluation of high-dose dexamethasone in strictly defined cerebral malaria, which showed that dexamethasone was deleterious (Warrell et al, 1982).

ANTI-MALARIAL DRUGS

Quinine

In the 1970s parenteral quinine doses as low as 5 mg (salt)/kg for 24 hours were being recommended for the treatment of severe falciparum malaria (Hall, 1976, 1977). These recommendations were based on studies which showed that serum concentrations of quinine in severe malaria were considerably higher than those measured in uncomplicated malaria or in volunteers. It was assumed, with very little evidence, that these total quinine concentrations (≥ 10 mg/l) were toxic. Indeed it has been the potential for toxicity, rather than a clear definition of the relationship between drug concentrations and effect, that has continued to limit quinine dosage. In acute falciparum malaria the total apparent volume of distribution (V_d) of quinine is contracted, and systemic clearance of the drug is reduced (White et al, 1982). These changes are directly proportional to disease severity and reflect increased protein binding (increased V_d; Silamut et al, 1991) and impaired liver, and to a lesser extent, renal, function (reduced clearance; White et al, 1982). Thus, for a given dose, plasma or whole blood quinine concentrations are higher in proportion to disease severity. The terminal elimination half-life is prolonged from approximately 11 hours in health to 18 hours in severe malaria. It takes approximately four half-lives for any drug to reach more than 90% of eventual steady-state blood or plasma concentrations, so for quinine the highest blood or plasma concentrations would be predicted after 3 or 4 days of treatment. But by this time the patient has usually either died or recovered. It is in the first 24–48 hours after admission to hospital that patients with severe malaria are at their greatest risk, and that most deaths occur. Thus, if a conventional dose regimen of 10 mg (salt)/kg every 8–12 hours is given without a loading dose, any risks associated with high plasma concentrations of quinine are incurred anyway (on the third or fourth day of treatment) without any of the benefits, but when the patient is at greatest risk from the malaria infection (i.e. within the first 24 hours), anti-malarial blood concentrations may be subtherapeutic (< 8–10 mg/l: White et al, 1983a). The reduced dose regimens recommended (i.e. < 10 mg/kg every 12 hours) ran a considerable risk of never achieving therapeutic concentrations. The obvious solution was to give an initial loading dose of quinine such that therapeutic concentrations would be achieved within 4 hours rather than the more than 24 hours with conventional dose regimens. This proved safe and effective (White et al, 1983a). Use of a quinine loading dose is now the recommended method of treating severe chloroquine-resistant falciparum malaria (WHO, 1986a, 1990).

The controversies that surround the use of a quinine loading dose have focused on potential toxicity. The argument runs that as blood or plasma concentration of quinine after a loading dose of 20 mg/kg are nearly twice those following a 'conventional' 10 mg/kg dose, the risks of toxicity should be greater. But as mentioned earlier, peak concentrations usually occur between the second and fourth days of treatment whether or not a loading dose is given. Thus, in the majority of patients blood or plasma quinine concentrations are lower immediately after the loading dose, than on the next day of treatment. In practice, with over 10 years of widespread use, the risks of toxicity are very low. Cardiotoxicity and neurotoxicity are the two principal serious adverse effects of quinine overdosage (Boland et al, 1985; Dyson et al, 1985). Cardiotoxicity is more pronounced with the dextro-rotatory stereoisomer quinidine (Phillips et al, 1985; Karbwang et al, 1993). Both hypotension (particularly if the drugs enter the circulation rapidly, such as following intravenous injection), and prolongation of repolarization (the 'quinidine effect') are dose related. Iatrogenic hypotension is very unusual with quinine, provided the drug is not given by intravenous injection. Quinidine has a four-fold greater effect on ventricular repolarization (prolongation of the electrocardiograph QT interval), compared with quinine although this is largely related to differences in plasma protein binding (Karbwang et al, 1993). However, even using quinidine with an initial loading dose, serious toxicity is very unusual (Phillips et al, 1985; Miller et al, 1989).

What is the therapeutic range for quinine? The upper limit is defined by toxicity and the lower limit by a suboptimal anti-malarial effect. Data on both are very limited. The symptom complex known as cinchonism consists of nausea, vomiting, dysphoria and tinnitus, and is a predictable accompaniment of quinine treatment. It appears with plasma concentrations over 5 mg/l, which in malaria correspond with free quinine concentrations of > 0.5 mg/l. Serious neurotoxicity is very unusual and consists of deafness and visual loss (Boland et al, 1985; Dyson et al, 1985). Although these serious neurotoxic reactions have been associated with plasma or serum quinine concentrations over 10 mg/l following self-poisoning in previously healthy adults, such concentrations are usual in the treatment of severe falciparum malaria, yet serious adverse effects are remarkably rare. In over 500 prospectively studied patients with severe falciparum malaria who were treated with a loading dose of parenteral quinine in Thailand and Viet Nam, there has not yet been one case of blindness, serious and persistent deafness, cardiac arrhythmia, significant (>25%) prolongation of the electrocardiograph QT_c interval, or definite iatrogenic hypotension (Pukrittayakamee et al, 1994). In those rare cases of blindness that have been reported in the treatment of malaria, total plasma quinine concentrations in many cases have not been unusually high. This suggests some idiosyncracy in the pharmacodynamic effect or unusually low plasma protein binding.

Much of the discrepancy between the incidence of toxicity following self-poisoning and that in severe malaria is explained by plasma protein binding (Silamut et al, 1991; Pukrittayakamee et al, 1994). Quinine is a basic drug which binds principally to α-1-acid-glycoprotein (orosomucoid). Blood concentrations of this acute phase protein are elevated markedly in trauma and sepsis, and severe malaria is no exception (Silamut et al, 1991). Thus plasma protein binding of quinine is increased in severe malaria, and the biologically active free fraction of the drug is correspondingly decreased. Plasma protein binding is increased from approximately 80% to over 90% (Silamut et al, 1991). Thus, the free fraction is reduced by half. By extrapolation from the very limited data available on plasma protein binding and the relationship between total quinine concentrations and toxicity in self-poisoning, it has been suggested recently that free plasma concentrations of quinine above 2 mg/l (corresponding to a total plasma concentration of > 20 mg/l) will be associated with an increased risk of toxicity (Winstanley et al, 1993). As quinine binding is pH dependent within the physiological range, and falls with the development of acidosis, patients with severe malaria may be at more risk of quinine toxicity than patients with uncomplicated disease. A loading dose of 15 mg (salt)/kg would be less likely to result in free plasma concentrations of over 2 mg/l, and it has been suggested that this dose might therefore be safer than the currently recommended loading dose of 20 mg (salt)/kg (Winstanley et al, 1993). This assumes that the risk of undertreatment is lower than that of toxicity. The argument would be easier to sustain if there was any evidence at all that initial doses of 20 mg/kg were associated with significant toxicity.

There have been four recent studies of quinine pharmacokinetics in African children with moderately severe or severe malaria (which is usually very sensitive to quinine in Africa) receiving a 20 mg/kg intramuscular or intravenous quinine loading dose. All have given similar results (Mansor et al, 1990; Waller et al, 1990; Pasvol et al, 1991; Winstanley et al, 1993). The risks of total plasma quinine concentrations exceeding 20 mg/l were 9% for intravenous administration and 20% for intramuscular administration. These risks would be reduced to 2% and 6.5%, respectively, by reducing the initial quinine dose to 15 mg/kg. But the price paid for this presumed increase in the margin of safety would be an increased risk that plasma concentrations of quinine in the critical first 12 hours of treatment would not exceed 5 mg/l. This plasma level (corresponding to a free concentration of 0.5 mg/l) has been shown in two trials to be associated with a submaximal therapeutic response (White et al, 1983a; Pasvol et al, 1991). With the modified (15 mg/kg) loading dose of quinine, this risk of potentially dangerous undertreatment rises from 0.2% to 3.8% for intravenous administration and from 2.0% to 10% for intramuscular administration. If no loading dose is given the risk that plasma concentrations do not exceed 5 mg/l in the first 8–12 hours (depending on dose interval) rises to 20.5% for intravenous and 30% for intramuscular administration. The true risks of undertreatment are not known because we do not know the shape of the in vivo dose–response curve. If a patient with severe malaria is untreated then they will usually die. Treatment regimens which result in mean total plasma quinine concentrations of ≤ 8 mg/l are associated with suboptimal therapeutic responses. Where this concentration lies on the dose-response curve is not known, but if it is on the steep part of the curve then lower plasma levels risk considerably less therapeutic effect. In an individual patient it is not possible to say, if the patient dies, that a larger dose of quinine would have been more effective. Our measures of therapeutic response in severe malaria (times to recovery, fever and parasite clearance etc.) are all taken over a longer time-span, and in any case refer to patients who survive, i.e. those who *are* adequately treated. Thus, the physician must balance an unknown risk of death from undertreatment, with a very low risk of serious (but rarely fatal) neurotoxicity or cardiovascular toxicity. We have argued (White and Krishna, 1989; Pukrittayakamee et al, 1992) that during the management of severe falciparum malaria the quinine risk/benefit ratio changes considerably. On admission the patient is at high risk of dying from malaria. Therapeutic levels of quinine should be reached as soon as safely possible (1–4 hours). Thereafter the risk/benefit ratio changes, and concern for toxicity becomes more prominent. If after 48 hours of treatment the patient's condition is not improved, or renal failure is established, then the doses of quinine should be reduced to avoid further accumulation of the drug. As the predominant route of quinine elimination is by hepatic biotransformation, liver dysfunction will also reduce clearance. In practice liver function usually improves with other clinical and laboratory indices. In ideal circumstances plasma concentrations should be measured as a guide to dosage, but this is rarely possible in the tropics, and the standard dose recommendations are nearly always both safe and effective.

Others have argued that the loading dose is unnecessary. 'Severe malaria responds perfectly well to quinine without using a loading dose'. It is true that the loading dose has never been proved unequivocally to reduce mortality, but then neither has any other treatment or drug regimen in severe malaria. Enormous sample sizes are required to show reductions in mortality with reasonable power. The largest comparative treatment studies in severe malaria ever to be conducted, which compare quinine loading dose regimens with intramuscular artemether, are now in progress. Before this there has never been a treatment comparison capable of detecting a reduction in mortality by anything less than 50%. Larger reductions in mortality with any treatment are unlikely as many patients die from severe malaria shortly after admission. These patients are probably beyond saving. Because of the wide variance in measures of the therapeutic response, such as the times to parasite clearance, fever clearance and coma recovery, large studies are required to show differences in these measures between two anti-malarial drug regimens, and in any case the relationship between these measures and a drug's life-saving potential is unclear (White and Krishna, 1989). The loading dose of quinine has never been subjected to a trial of sufficient size to define its benefits clearly. These can only be extrapolated indirectly from the arguments given earlier (Pukrittayakamee et al, 1992). Those trials reported have indicated benefit (Fargier et al, 1991; Pasvol et al, 1991; Pukrittayakamee et al, 1992). Other life-saving drugs with long elimination half-lives are usually given in an initial loading dose and there is no justification for excluding quinine from this general pharmacological principle. As with the other controversies and areas of disagreement which follow, recommendations have commonly been based on anecdotal personal experience (of very limited statistical power), or extrapolations from incorrect pathophysiological assumptions. The use of a quinine loading dose has been based on sound pharmacological principles, some evidence of benefit, and it has not been associated with increased risks to patients.

Many patients with severe malaria have received quinine before they are admitted to hospital. Although there have been recent developments which may allow rapid assessment of quinine concentrations in blood, these are not available widely. Indirect assessments based on high-tone hearing (Roche et al, 1990; Karlsson et al, 1990) or the QT prolongation on the electrocardiogram (White et al, 1983b) are insufficiently precise. If patients are admitted with therapeutic concentrations of quinine already present in the blood, then a loading dose is clearly unnecessary, and certainly would be potentially dangerous. We do not give a loading dose if there is a clear history that more than 2 g of quinine have been given in the previous 48 hours. Even though the history is notoriously unreliable in such cases, we have not encountered toxicity using this general treatment guide-line.

Intramuscular quinine

Quinine dihydrochloride, the usual parenteral formulation (300 mg/ml), has a pH of 2. In experimental animals intramuscular injection produces necrosis and sterile abscess formation (Ross, 1914; Fletcher and Visuvalingam, 1923). In the treatment of falciparum malaria intramuscular quinine has been associated with abscess formation and sometimes disfiguring secondary scarring, sciatic nerve damage and tetanus (Yen et al, 1994). Although widely used throughout this century, as mentioned previously many leading authorities have argued against the intramuscular route of administration (Ross, 1914). However, in much of the rural tropics, this is the only feasible approach to the treatment of severe malaria. After a period of contradictory recommendations (WHO, 1986b), in the past few years a consensus has emerged that intramuscular quinine is an acceptable treatment for severe falciparum malaria in rural areas where slow intravenous infusions cannot be managed adequately (WHO, 1986a, 1990). The complication rate in terms of severe pain or abscess formation following undiluted quinine can be reduced considerably by the use of careful aseptic technique, injection only into the anterior thigh, and not the buttock, and vigorous massaging after the injection has been given. In Papua New Guinea a dilute formulation (60 mg (salt)/ml) has been widely used for over 15 years without apparent complications (Adelusi et al, 1982). Following intramuscular injection, quinine is well absorbed with a bio-availability of over 85% (Mansor et al, 1990; Waller et al, 1990; Pasvol et al, 1991; Pukrittayakamee et al, 1992; Winstanley et al, 1993). Plasma concentration profiles are similar to those with intravenous infusions (Pukrittayakamee et al, 1992). The optimum pharmacokinetic properties are associated with the undiluted, more acidic, and more locally toxic concentration (Pasvol et al, 1991). However, dilute formulations are absorbed more rapidly than undiluted solutions (usually 300 mg/ml: Waller et al, 1990) and the risk that dangerously rapid absorption may occur leading to hypotension, analagous to that following intramuscular chloroquine, is increased. These risks have not been quantified. The optimum concentration of quinine for intramuscular injection remains to be determined.

Parenteral chloroquine

When the World Health Organization announced that parenteral chloroquine should no longer be used because of its potential toxicity (WHO, 1984), chloroquine was the most widely used anti-malarial drug for the treatment of severe malaria, and was probably the second most prescribed of any drug in the world. This recommendation was based on several anecdotal reports of sudden death following intramuscular chloroquine administration to children. The incidence of these fatal reactions was not known at that time as there had been no pharmacokinetic studies of chloroquine in severe malaria. It was shown subsequently that chloroquine was absorbed very rapidly after intramuscular or subcutaneous injections, reaching peak blood concentrations within 10–30 minutes (Gustafsson et al, 1983; White et al, 1987, 1988a). Although the terminal elimination half-life of chloroquine is extremely long (1–2 months) and the total apparent volume distribution is enormous (100–1000 l/kg: White et al, 1987), the central compartment into which chloroquine distributes initially is considerably smaller (Looareesuwan et al, 1986). As it takes hours or days for chloroquine to equilibrate in the body by binding to various tissues, it is distribution rather than elimination processes that govern the blood concentration profile (White, 1992). As a consequence, after intramuscular or subcutaneous injection (or intravenous injection), chloroquine enters the blood stream much faster than it can leave it, and transiently high and potentially toxic blood concentrations are reached. These may cause hypotension, and probably account for the occasional sudden death that followed treatment with intramuscular or subcutaneous chloroquine. Intravenous injections of chloroquine are dangerous and should not be used (Looareesuwan et al, 1986). The risks of parenteral chloroquine may have been exacerbated by the common practice of administering a single intramuscular injection of chloroquine to a young and seriously ill child, who is then discharged immediately from the clinic (White et al, 1987). As many of these babies are carried upright on their mothers' backs there is also a postural component to the hypotension. This may also have accounted for the sudden deaths that prompted the 1984 advice against chloroquine (WHO, 1984). The solution to these problems was to give smaller and more frequent doses of intramuscular or subcutaneous chloroquine (i.e. treatment with 5 mg (base)/kg every 6 hours, or 2.5 mg (base)/kg every 4 hours), and to give intravenous chloroquine by constant rate infusion. With these regimens transient dangerous blood chloroquine concentrations do not occur (White et al, 1988a). Unfortunately, although chloroquine may be superior to quinine (White et al, 1989), probably because of its action at an earlier stage in the intraerythrocytic parasite life cycle, there are now few countries in the tropics where chloroquine can be relied upon as a first-line treatment for severe falciparum malaria.

Artemisinin and its derivatives: which drug?

Since the discovery of the anti-malarial properties of extracts of the plant qinghao by the Chinese in 1971, several derivatives of the parent compound (artemisinin: qinghaosu) have been developed (Qinghaosu Antimalaria Coordinating Group, 1979). These are the water-soluble hemisuccinate derivate, artesunate, and the oil-soluble ethers, artemether and arteether (Hien and White, 1993). All of these, and the parent compound artemisinin, are converted to a common biologically active metabolite, dihydroartemisinin (Lee and Hufford, 1990). This has recently become available in tablet formulation. In addition a structurally related peroxide derived from the plant yinghaozu has been developed recently for oral use (artiflene). Progress in developing and evaluating these compounds has been slow, and there is still considerable disagreement over the correct strategy for the immediate future.

The compounds available in 1994 for the treatment of severe malaria were artemisinin in suppository formulation (available only in Viet Nam), artesunate for intramuscular and intravenous administration, artemether for intramuscular administration only and, currently under clinical trial, arteether (also for intramuscular administration). Artesunate and artemether have been used extensively over the past 10 years in the treatment of severe malaria. They have proved rapidly effective, indeed they appear to be the most rapidly effective of all anti-malarial drugs, and there has been no evident toxicity in man (Hien and White, 1993). However, because both these compounds were produced in factories which at the time did not comply with international standards of 'Good Manufacturing Practices', and because the information dossiers on these compounds were insufficient to obtain regulatory approval in Western countries, the World Health Organization decided in 1984 to embark on the development of arteether (Davidson, 1994). The objective of this course was to develop the compound through internationally accepted processes of standard manufacture, pre-clinical testing and, eventually, clinical evaluation such that it would obtain regulatory approval and a well-tested, well-certified compound would be available generally at a low price. Ten years later, arteether has just entered preliminary clinical trials in uncomplicated malaria. Meanwhile the dossier of information on artemether, and the manufacturing processes, have both improved to the point where international regulatory approval is anticipated and an acceptable pharmaceutical product is already available for the treatment of severe malaria (Roche and Helenport, 1994). Artesunate, the most widely used, and considered by many to be the most effective of all the compounds, languishes on the regulatory rocks. The parenteral formulation is not produced to the standards required by Good Manufacturing Practices, and would not therefore meet international regulatory requirements.

The compounds available

Artesunate is intrinsically unstable. It is supplied for parenteral use as a powder of artesunic acid together with an ampoule of 5% sodium bicarbonate. The two are mixed immediately before intramuscular or intravenous injection. Conversion to the biologically active metabolite dihydroartemisinin happens almost instantaneously once the drugs enter the circulation (and probably also occurs in the syringe!). Despite the fact that parenteral artesunate does not meet international regulatory requirements and is not produced to Good Manufacturing Practices standards, it is very widely used and there have been no reports of serious toxicity. Artemether *is* now available in an acceptable pharmaceutical formulation, but it may only be given by intramuscular injection, and therefore the speed of onset of anti-malarial action is determined by the rate of absorption after intramuscular injection. This probably explains why it is slightly slower acting than parenteral artesunate (White, 1994), a difference that may be clinically important in the treatment of fulminant malaria. In addition the oil-soluble ethers have produced an unusual, but reproducible, pattern of neurotoxicity in experimental animals (Brewer et al, 1994). This involves selective damage to brain stem nuclei and, although it has occurred at doses somewhat higher than those used in the treatment of severe malaria, these observations have given rise to considerable concern. However, there is no evidence yet that similar toxicity occurs in man with currently recommended dose regimens. The common metabolite dihydroartemisinin (DHA) induces the same pattern of neurotoxicity. This would suggest that all compounds are equally neurotoxic (as all are metabolized to DHA), but in the experimental animals the water-soluble drugs were less neurotoxic. Arteether differs from artemether simply by the substitution of an ethyl for a methyl group. There seems to be no significant differences between the two compounds, although arteether has yet to be used for the treatment of severe malaria, whereas artemether has been used in over 100 000 patients. Six large trials comparing artemether and quinine in the treatment of severe malaria will finish in 1994. These should allow a confident assessment of the relative merits of the two compounds, but where will this leave arteether? From a regulatory standpoint this is a different compound from artemether and therefore it cannot be assumed that any advantages or disadvantages that are demonstrated in the clinical trials would also obtain with arteether. Unless similar large studies are conducted to define the role of arteether we will be left in the position of having a compound which is very similar to the established one, but not identical, with uncertain efficacy and toxicity. Many have questioned the wisdom of continuing to invest a considerable proportion of the meagre funds available for anti-malarial drug development to a compound almost identical to one already available.

Artemisinin suppositories have been shown in comparative studies to be equally efficacious in terms of clinical and parasitological responses to the parenteral artemisinin derivatives (Arnold et al, 1990; Hien et al, 1992). These are produced in Viet Nam and are not available elsewhere. Artesunate suppositories, and intrarectal artemether are also being evaluated. The comparative trials with these drugs, as with all other published trials to date, have been of insufficient power to detect anything other than large differences between compounds and formulations. However, this method of drug administration is of great potential. A suppository formulation would have considerable advantages for the treatment of severe malaria in the rural tropics as it would extend the usage to the village level (WHO, 1993). Suppositories also avoid the obvious dangers of needle use and can be administered by otherwise unqualified people.

The asynchronous development of these compounds and the slowly emerging evidence on efficacy and safety has resulted in the peculiar situation that most of the limited available funding and support is going to arteether (which in 1994 has yet to be given to a patient with severe malaria), and to a lesser extent artemether (an almost identical compound), while we know relatively little about artesunate, which appears to be safer and more effective and is by far the most widely used drug. For example at the time of writing we know considerably more about the pharmacokinetic properties of arteether in dogs than of any of the artemisinin derivatives in humans with malaria. There are no reliable pharmacokinetic data on any of the currently available drugs from patients with severe malaria.

The next question is where should these drugs be used? The general consensus is that until artemisinin or its derivatives have been shown un-equivocally to be intrinsically superior to quinine (i.e. to reduce mortality in an area with fully quinine-sensitive falciparum malaria or to be safer), their use should be restricted to areas with significant quinine resistance (WHO, 1993). In practice this means the drugs should not be used in Africa until they have been proved to be superior to quinine there. Quinine resist-ance is already a problem in South America and South East Asia, and there the drugs have a real place as alternatives to quinine, but whether they reduce mortality or not, and which drugs should be used, remains to be determined.

ANTI-MALARIAL TREATMENT: THE QUALITY OF EVIDENCE

The choice of treatment for severe malaria depends on scientific evidence and clinical experience. How do we make our decisions? The overall mortality reported for cerebral malaria is approximately 20%. Thus, in order to detect a reduction in mortality by 25% with 95% confidence and 80% power, a comparative trial must include approximately 1000 patients in each treatment arm. No trial in severe malaria has gone anywhere near this sample size. Comparative trials in the past have therefore used other measures of the therapeutic response, in the hope that these would also reflect a similar effect on mortality or, more recently, have endeavoured to detect differences in mortality of a larger magnitude (i.e. 33–50% reductions in mortality). The other measures of the therapeutic responses that have been used in severe malaria treatment comparisons can be justified as described below.

Time to recovery of consciousness in cerebral malaria

It is reasonable to assume that the processes that cause coma also cause death, at least in a proportion of the patients. In addition patients who remain unconscious for longer are more prone to secondary complications such as aspiration pneumonia, spontaneous septicaemia, etc.

Time to fever clearance

Fever in malaria is related to the release of pyrogenic cytokines. Levels of tumour necrosis factor (TNF) are increased considerably in fatal cases (Grau et al, 1989; Kwiatkowski et al, 1990), and it has been suggested that high levels of TNF may kill patients with severe malaria, although this is unproven. Cytokines are produced when malaria 'toxins' are released at schizont rupture. Drugs which reduce the duration of fever presumably attenuate either the production or the response to malaria pyrogens, and may therefore be beneficial by interrupting these processes.

Parasite clearance times

The prognosis in severe malaria is directly related to the parasite burden. The peripheral blood parasitaemia is an imprecise reflection of the total parasite burden. This relationship is confounded by the sequestration of red cells containing mature, pathogenic forms of the parasite in the micro-vasculature. Thus the microscopist does not count the parasites causing the most harm (Silamut and White, 1993). Nevertheless, persistence of parasites in the peripheral blood (area under the parasitaemia–time curve) is related to the parasite burden, and certainly failure to clear parasitaemia reflects resistance of the infection to the anti-malarial treatment. Indeed, because of the 48 hour parasite cycle, the proportional reduction in parasitaemia/cycle (parasite reduction ratio) can be used as an in vivo pharmacodynamic measure of anti-malarial drug effect. This is because parasites persisting beyond 48 hours after starting anti-malarial treatment largely represent a generation that has emerged in the presence of the drug. Thus, increasing parasite clearance times are a sensitive reflection of drug resistance and a useful comparative measure in uncomplicated and severe malaria drug trials. There is some debate about the relative merits of measuring the times to 50%, 90%, 95%, 99% or 100% clearance. Times to 50% clearance really reflect the efficacy of the anti-malarial in accelerating ring-form clearance, whereas times to 100% clearance can be distorted by counting errors and the continued detection of small pyknotic, probably dead, intraerythrocytic parasites.

The recrudescence rates after anti-malarial treatment are of secondary concern in severe malaria as the primary objective of treatment is to save life. It is worth reiterating that none of these measures has been proved a good surrogate of life-saving efficacy.

Bias

Although there have been no large definitive comparative treatment studies in severe malaria, there have been many small or open studies, and an unusually high proportion of these have had positive results. The problems of bias in open studies are well-known and the results of these studies should be interpreted with caution and in the context of other reported experience.

RAISED INTRACRANIAL PRESSURE

Cerebral oedema has been widely considered as a primary pathological process in fatal cerebral malaria. This led to the evaluation of various measures to reduce cerebral oedema including use of urea, mannitol and high-dose corticosteroids. However, several lines of evidence argue against a consistent role for cerebral oedema in the pathogenesis of cerebral malaria. These may be summarized as follows:

1. Computerized tomography and magnetic resonance imaging both show that the brain is not usually oedematous in vivo (Looareesuwan et al, 1983; Newton et al, 1994), contrary to recent predictions (Poser and Roman, 1991).
2. Papilloedema is not common in cerebral malaria (Davis et al, 1992; Lewallen et al, 1993).
3. In the original simian models that showed high-dose corticosteroids to reverse increased blood–brain barrier permeability (Maegraith and Fletcher, 1972), chloroquine was shown to have the same action, yet chloroquine is not effective treatment for cerebral malaria caused by chloroquine-resistant strains of *P. falciparum.*
4. Two double-blind comparative trials have shown no benefit from high-dose corticosteroids (Warrell et al, 1982; Hoffman et al, 1988). In the largest of these, high-dose corticosteroids were also associated with an increased incidence of infective complications.
5. Studies of blood–brain barrier permeability in cerebral malaria do not indicate an increase in permeability. The increased influx and efflux of ^{125}I labelled albumin shown in the original simian models were not confirmed in man (Warrell et al, 1986).

As a consequence of these observations high-dose corticosteroids are considered contra-indicated in cerebral malaria. This is not to say that cerebral oedema *never* occurs, but that it is a relatively uncommon and inconsistent feature. However, the role of raised intracranial pressure and possible brain stem coning as a lethal event in cerebral malaria remains an unresolved and important area for further study (Newton et al, 1991). Although in 80% of adult cases of cerebral malaria the opening pressure at lumbar puncture is within the normal range (Warrell et al, 1986), only 20% of children with cerebral malaria have normal lumbar puncture opening pressures (Newton et al, 1991; Waller et al, 1991; White, 1991). In fact, the mean pressures in both adults and children are similar (around 160 mm of CSF), but because the normal range in children is much lower this means that about 80% of children have raised pressures. Provided that there is no obstruction to cerebrospinal fluid flow, lumbar puncture opening pressure should reflect intracranial pressure. In general this is true but the measurement of lumbar puncture opening pressure at a single time point has been shown to be a poor reflection of maximum intracranial pressures measured directly by a pressure transducer inserted through the skull into the extradural space (Newton et al, 1994). Children with cerebral malaria have been shown to have paroxysmal marked rises in intracranial pressure which in some cases have been sufficient to compromise cerebral perfusion (Newton et al, 1994). Furthermore, it has been argued that the brain stem signs commonly observed in cerebral malaria reflect the development of a tentorial or foramen magnum pressure cone (Newton et al, 1991). As a result of these observations it has been suggested that lumbar puncture may be dangerous in childhood cerebral malaria, and should be delayed. Some groups prefer to give empirical chloramphenicol to 'cover' meningitis and then to perform a lumbar puncture on recovery from coma. On the other hand it has been argued that lumbar puncture opening pressures are not significantly different in fatal cases and survivors (White, 1991), that there is no evidence that lumbar puncture is harmful (by precipitating fatal coning), and that the brain stem signs attributed to coning are common in survivors. Most authorities still recommend early lumbar puncture in cerebral malaria as they consider that the risks of undiagnosed meningitis outweigh the undefined potential harm from lumbar puncture in suspected cerebral malaria. The chances of a wrong diagnosis increase with inexperience of the medical practitioners and so may be inversely proportional to the quality of care.

The cause of raised intracranial pressure in cerebral malaria is probably an increase in the intracerebral blood volume, resulting from intracerebral sequestration of parasitized erythrocytes and compensatory vasodilatation to maintain cerebral perfusion (Looareesuwan et al, 1995). Although there may be some increase in capillary permeability related to this process, this does not lead to significant oedema in vivo. The most likely explanation for the paroxysmal changes in intracranial pressure that have been recorded are changes in vascular tone. The critical and unresolved question is how commonly these paroxysmal rises of intracranial pressure are either sufficient to reduce cerebral perfusion to the degree that infarction occurs, or are unevenly distributed and lead to the development of a fatal pressure cone. The clinical progression of brain stem signs leading to respiratory arrest would certainly be consistent with such a diagnosis but these signs are also common in survivors. The differential diagnosis is therefore between intrinsic brain stem pathology causing respiratory arrest, or extrinsic pressure. The relationship between intracranial pressure, cerebral perfusion and function, and risk of fatal coning is inconsistent. For example, in cryptococcal meningitis lumbar puncture opening pressures may be considerably higher than those usually recorded in cerebral malaria, and may be sustained for weeks in some cases, with a low risk of fatal coning. This presumably reflects an even distribution of pressure change and raises the question of why an apparently diffuse process such as intracranial sequestration in falciparum malaria should lead to differential pressure changes sufficient to cause downward displacement of the brain stem. Potentially lethal downward displacement of the brain stem has been observed in two magnetic resonance imaging scans from adults who died from cerebral malaria, but in both of these the scans were taken after respiratory arrest and resuscitation, so whether they were a cause or a result of this event cannot be determined (Looareesuwan et al, 1995). Pathological evidence of brain stem compression at autopsy of fatal cases of adult cerebral malaria is unusual. There are insufficient data from published autopsy findings in children. The question remains open.

There may be significant differences between adults and children in intracranial pathology in cerebral malaria. Whilst cerebral oedema does not appear to play a primary role in pathogenesis, raised intracranial pressure is commonly found in childhood cerebral malaria and may be of sufficient degree to compromise cerebral perfusion. Fatal coning may occur, but it is not possible at the present time to say how commonly this is the terminal event, nor whether therapeutic strategies aimed at reducing intracranial pressure would benefit children with cerebral malaria. Mannitol is undoubtedly effective and would be a logical therapy, but in the absence of further information on the pharmacokinetics and pharmacodynamics of mannitol in childhood cerebral malaria, and without clinical evidence of benefit or an evaluation of potential adverse effects, it would seem premature to recommend use of this or other osmotic agents in the treatment of cerebral malaria. Hopefully clinical trials will resolve these uncertainties.

OTHER ADJUNCTIVE THERAPIES

There is a long list of drugs or other substances that have been recommended as adjunctive therapies in severe falciparum malaria.

In addition to osmotic agents such as mannitol, urea and glycerol, and the high-dose corticosteroids mentioned previously, low molecular mass dextran, heparin, prostacyclin, oxpentifylline, aspirin, N-acetyl-cysteine, desferrioxamine, anti-TNF antibody, anti-malarial immunoglobulin, phenobarbitone and dichloroacetate have all been suggested. The use of heparin was popular in the 1970s when disseminated intravascular coagulation was considered an important pathophysiological mechanism in many serious diseases. This was associated with an unusually high incidence of severe bleeding (Punyagupta et al, 1974) and is no longer recommended. Aspirin has also been shown recently to be of no benefit (Hemmer et al, 1991).

Prophylactic anticonvulsants

Convulsions are common in children and seem to be associated with both an increased mortality and neurological deficit (Molyneux et al, 1989; Brewster et al, 1990). A very small dose of intramuscular phenobarbitone has been shown to reduce the incidence of convulsions in adults (White et al, 1988b). However, the incidence of convulsions in adults with cerebral malaria varies considerably. For example, in Thailand it has fallen from 50% to less than 20% over the past 10 years without any obvious explanation. In children, where the incidence is higher, the optimum dose or choice of anti-convulsant remains to be determined. Pharmacokinetic data (ter Kuile et al, 1992; Winstanley et al, 1992) suggest that conventional loading doses of phenobarbitone should be used (i.e. around 15 mg/kg) but there are insufficient pharmacodynamic data (i.e. on the level of sedation or recovery of consciousness) for a firm recommendation to be made.

Although anti-pyretics are used almost universally in the treatment of cerebral malaria, it has been argued that a high fever may be beneficial by inhibiting schizont development and possibly by potentiating neutrophil function. Balanced against this is the increase in metabolic rate (particularly of the brain) in fever which would exacerbate the supply and demand imbalance in the sequestered microcirculation. In addition high fever lowers the seizure threshold, a particular problem in young children.

Dichloracetate

Dichloracetate has been suggested as a specific treatment for lactic acidosis in severe falciparum malaria (Holloway et al, 1991). It has not proved effective in other causes of lactic acidosis, although it has been argued that in the other conditions in which it has been used the causes of death were multifactorial and that amelioration of lactic acidosis would not have been expected to alter the natural history of the disease. Dichloroacetate has proved effective in a rodent model of severe malaria (Holloway et al, 1991). Lactic acidosis is undoubtedly an important pathophysiological process in severe falciparum malaria and dichloroacetate has been shown to reduce hyperlactataemia in recent studies (Krishna et al, 1994). Clinical trials to determine whether mortality can be reduced are planned.

Anti-TNF antibody

Anti-TNF antibody reduced fever in children with cerebral malaria (Kwiatkowski et al, 1993) and a large double-blind placebo controlled study of anti-TNF antibody is currently in progress. There are many different anti-TNF antibodies each with different affinities, avidities and neutralizing potencies. Until the results of this are available it would seem premature to recommend this expensive treatment.

Desferrioxamine

Desferrioxamine has been shown to reduce significantly the duration of coma in Zambian children with cerebral malaria in a double-blind placebo controlled study (Gordeuk et al, 1992). Desferrioxamine has two potentially beneficial actions: the first is an anti-malarial effect which is slow and analagous to that of the anti-malarial antibiotics (Gordeuk et al, 1993); the second, which is of particular relevance to cerebral malaria, is a specific anti-oxidant effect that might be cytoprotective. Although this was a well conducted trial, the duration of coma in the placebo group was significantly longer than that usually reported in African children with cerebral malaria, while the duration of coma in the desferrioxamine group was similar to that observed elsewhere. It should also be noted that in vitro desferrioxamine antagonizes the anti-malarial effects of artemisinin and its derivatives.

Thus, of the many adjunctive therapies mentioned, only anti-convulsants and anti-pyretics are currently recommended.

VENTILATION

As respiratory arrest appears to be a common cause of death, particularly in children with cerebral malaria, it would seem reasonable for patients to be ventilated electively. This would be of potential benefit either to sustain ventilation through intrinsic but hopefully reversible brain stem pathology, or by maintaining hypocapnia and thus reducing intracranial pressure and preventing external brain stem compression (although recent opinion is divided on the dangers of reducing cerebral perfusion and adversely affecting outcome). It could be argued that patients with lactic acidosis and an appropriate respiratory drive would maintain a lower intracranial pressure as a result of hyperventilation and hypocapnia. If the respiratory drive were reduced in cerebral malaria, then intracranial pressure might rise and, if this were unevenly distributed, lead to coning. These arguments are all linked with the previous debate over the role of intracranial pressure and the pathology of brain stem dysfunction in cerebral malaria. It should be noted that the optimum arterial P_{CO_2} value to aim for in cerebral malaria is not known. In the absence of further information it would seem reasonable to ventilate patients showing respiratory abnormalities provided adequate nursing facilities were available and to maintain the P_{CO_2} at approximately 4 to 4.5 kPa (30–35 mmHg). Now that is all very well in adequately staffed and equipped intensive care units, but as the world distribution of such intensive care units is inversely proportional to the distribution of severe malaria, the two coincide relatively infrequently.

DIALYSIS

Acute renal failure in severe falciparum malaria results from acute tubular necrosis, and develops in one of three interconnected circumstances:

1. Multisystem dysfunction in the acute phase of fulminant malaria.
2. Following severe malaria.
3. Associated with massive haemoglobinuria.

After adequate rehydration, preferably guided by central venous pressure measurement, the decision on 'when to dialyse' is based on several considerations. Obviously dialysis should be undertaken immediately if there is hyperkalaemia (rare in malaria), fluid overload, uraemic symptoms or signs, or unresponsive acidosis. In general it is best to dialyse early in situation 1 above, i.e. in fulminant disease. Haemofiltration or haemodialysis will regain metabolic control faster than peritoneal dialysis, but they are seldom available. There is no easy rule of thumb, but serum creatinine concentrations over 400 μmol/l are usually associated with a need to dialyse in this context. In situations 2 and 3 above, there is less urgency and, particularly if facilities are limited, the physician can afford to wait a little if urine flow is maintained. The patient should be examined frequently, the serum potassium checked twice daily and if blood transfusion is required, it should be given very slowly. It is not uncommon for patients with subacute presentations of acute renal failure who are not oliguric to have serum creatinine concentrations rise as high as 600–800 μmol/l and then 'turn the corner' and recover. In most patients dialysis will not be required for more than 4–5 days, but some will require 2–3 weeks. The management is that of acute renal failure in any setting. Infections are common and there is usually considerable weight loss.

EXCHANGE TRANSFUSION

In malaria, pathology results from the parasitization of erythrocytes. Therefore in patients with very high parasitaemias, why not remove as many of the infected cells as possible, and replace them by uninfected ones? The best and quickest way to do this is by exchange transfusion and, although this has never been subjected to controlled clinical trials, a number of anecdotal reports and a small series do suggest that exchange transfusion may be of benefit (Looareesuwan et al, 1990). This begs the question as to how it works. Obviously exchange transfusion will only remove those red cells that are circulating, and yet the circulating parasitized erythrocytes are not thought to be those that are causing harm. It is the sequestered red cells containing mature parasites that are thought to be pathological. Perhaps it is the noxious substances in plasma rather than the red cells themselves that are harmful? There is even one report of plasma exchange being beneficial. Obviously young ring-form infected erythrocytes will develop into more pathological mature sequestering forms if anti-malarial treatment is not effective and, certainly in the case of quinine which acts only on the more mature parasites, this would be another argument in support of exchange transfusion. A carefully controlled clinical trial would help to resolve these issues. Currently a pragmatic solution to these uncertainties would be to employ exchange transfusion if facilities and cross-matched virus-free blood were available. Indications for exchange transfusion are also unclear. It has been recommended that exchange transfusion should be conducted if there is more than 15% parasitaemia, and should be considered for parasitaemias between 5% and 15% if there is other evidence of vital organ dysfunction. The use of artemisinin derivatives in severe malaria may reduce the indications for exchange transfusion as they reduce parasitaemia much more rapidly than other anti-malarials.

SUMMARY

As most cases of severe malaria are managed in rural areas where there are limited health care facilities, the real challenge is to introduce improvements that are readily and safely applicable in these circumstances. It is there that the greatest impact is likely to be made. Prevention of malaria, or early recognition of potentially life-threatening disease, is likely to save many more lives than the treatment of severe infections.

REFERENCES

Adelusi SA, Dawodu AH & Salako LA (1982) Kinetics of the uptake and elimination of chloroquine in children with malaria. *British Journal of Clinical Pharmacology* 14: 483–487.

Arnold K, Hien TT, Nguyen TC et al (1990) A randomized comparative study of artemisinine (qinghaosu) suppositories and oral quinine in acute falciparum malaria. *Transactions of the Royal Society of Tropical Medicine and Hygiene* 84: 499–502.

Boland ME, Roper SM & Henry JA (1985) Complications of quinine poisoning. *Lancet* i: 384–385.

Brewer TG, Peggins JO, Grate SJ et al (1994) Neurotoxicity in animals due to arteether and artemether. *Transactions of the Royal Society of Tropical Medicine and Hygiene* 88 (supplement 1): 33–36.

Brewster DR, Kwiatkowski D & White NJ (1990) Neurological sequelae of cerebral malaria in children. *Lancet* 336: 1039–1043.

Davidson DE Jr (1994) Role of arteether in the treatment of malaria and plans for further development. *Transactions of the Royal Society of Tropical Medicine and Hygiene* 88 (supplement 1): 51–52.

Davis TME, Supanaranond W, Spencer JL et al (1992) Measures of capillary permeability in acute falciparum malaria: relation to severity of infection and treatment. *Clinical Infectious Diseases* 15: 256–266.

Dyson EH, Proudfoot AT, Prescott LF & Heyworth R (1985) Death and blindness due to overdose of quinine. *British Medical Journal* 291: 31–33.

Fargier JJ, Louis FJ, Cot M et al (1991) Reduction of coma by quinine loading dose in falciparum cerebral malaria. *Lancet* 338: 896–897 (letter).

Fletcher W & Visuvalingam SA (1923) Intramuscular injections of quinine. In Fletcher W (ed.) *Studies from the Institute for Medical Research, Kuala Lumpur, Federated Malay States. Notes on the Treatment of Malaria with Alkaloids of Cinchona*, pp 24–42. London: John Bale & Sons and Danielsson.

Gordeuk V, Thuma P, Brittenham G et al (1992) Effect of iron chelation therapy on recovery from deep coma in children with cerebral malaria. *New England Journal of Medicine* 327: 1473–1477 (see comments).

Gordeuk VR, Thuma PE, Brittenham GM et al (1993) Iron chelation as a chemotherapeutic strategy for falciparum malaria. *American Journal of Tropical Medicine and Hygiene* **48:** 193–197.

Grau GE, Taylor TE, Molyneux ME et al (1989) Tumor necrosis factor and disease severity in children with falciparum malaria. *New England Journal of Medicine* **320:** 1586–1591.

Gustafsson LL, Walker O, Alvan G et al (1983) Disposition of chloroquine in man after single intravenous and oral doses. *British Journal of Clinical Pharmacology* **15:** 471–479.

Hall AP (1976) The treatment of malaria. *British Medical Journal* **1:** 323–328.

Hall AP (1977) The treatment of severe falciparum malaria. *Transactions of the Royal Society of Tropical Medicine and Hygiene* **71:** 367–378.

Hemmer CJ, Kern P, Holst FG et al (1991) Neither heparin nor acetylsalicylic acid influence the clinical course in human *Plasmodium falciparum* malaria: a prospective randomized study. *American Journal of Tropical Medicine and Hygiene* **45:** 608–612.

Hien TT & White NJ (1993) Qinghaosu. *Lancet* **341:** 603–608.

Hien TT, Arnold K, Vinh H et al (1992) Comparison of artemisinin suppositories with intravenous artesunate and intravenous quinine in the treatment of cerebral malaria. *Transactions of the Royal Society of Tropical Medicine and Hygiene* **86:** 582–583.

Hoffman SL, Rustama D, Punjabi NH et al (1988) High-dose dexamethasone in quinine-treated patients with cerebral malaria: a double-blind, placebo-controlled trial. *Journal of Infectious Diseases* **158:** 325–331.

Holloway PA, Krishna S & White NJ (1991) *Plasmodium berghei*: lactic acidosis and hypoglycaemia in a rodent model of severe malaria, effects of glucose, quinine, and dichloroacetate. *Experimental Parasitology* **72:** 123–133.

Karbwang J, Davis TME, Looareesuwan S et al (1993) A comparison of the pharmacokinetic and pharmacodynamic properties of quinine and quinidine in healthy Thai males. *British Journal of Clinical Pharmacology* **35:** 265–271.

Karlsson KK, Hellgren U, Alvan G & Rombo L (1990) Audiometry as a possible indicator of quinine plasma concentration during treatment and of malaria. *Transactions of the Royal Society of Tropical Medicine and Hygiene* **84:** 765–767.

Krishna S, Supanaranond W, Pukrittayakamee S et al (1994) Dichloroacetate for lactic acidosis in severe malaria: a pharmacokinetic and pharmacodynamic assessment. *Metabolism* **43:** 974–981.

Kwiatkowski D, Hill AVS, Sambou I et al (1990) TNF concentrations in fatal cerebral, non-fatal cerebral, and uncomplicated *Plasmodium falciparum* malaria. *Lancet* **336:** 1201–1204.

Kwiatkowski D, Molyneux ME, Stephens S et al (1993) Anti-TNF therapy inhibits fever in cerebral malaria. *Quarterly Journal Medicine* **86:** 91–98.

Lee IS & Hufford CD (1990) Metabolism of antimalarial sesquiterpene lactones. *Pharmacology and Therapeutics* **48:** 345–355.

Lewallen S, Taylor TE, Molyneux ME et al (1993) Ocular fundus findings in Malawian children with cerebral malaria. *Ophthalmology* **100:** 857–861.

Looareesuwan S, Warrell DA, White NJ et al (1983a) Do patients with cerebral malaria have cerebral oedema? A computed tomography study. *Lancet* **i:** 434–437.

Looareesuwan S, White NJ, Chanthavanich P et al (1986) Cardiovascular toxicity and distribution kinetics of intravenous chloroquine. *British Journal of Clinical Pharmacology* **22:** 31–36.

Looareesuwan S, Phillips RE, Karbwang J et al (1990) *Plasmodium falciparum* hyperparasitaemia: use of exchange transfusion in seven patients and a review of the literature. *Quarterly Journal of Medicine* **75:** 471–481.

Looareesuwan S, Wilairatana P, Krishna S et al (1995) Magnetic resonance imaging of the brain in cerebral malaria. *Clinical Infectious Diseases* (in the press).

Maegraith B & Fletcher A (1972) The pathogenesis of mammalian malaria. *Advances in Parasitology* **10:** 49–75.

Mansor SM, Taylor TE, McGrath CS et al (1990) The safety and kinetics of intramuscular quinine in Malawian children with moderately severe falciparum malaria. *Transactions of the Royal Society of Tropical Medicine and Hygiene* **84:** 482–487.

Miller KD, Greenberg AE & Campbell CC (1989) Treatment of severe malaria in the United States with a continuous infusion of quinidine gluconate and exchange transfusion. *New England Journal of Medicine* **321:** 65–70.

Molyneux ME, Taylor TE, Wirima JJ & Borgstein J (1989) Clinical features and prognostic indicators in paediatric cerebral malaria: a study of 131 comatose Malawian children. *Quarterly Journal of Medicine* **71:** 441–459.

Newton CRJC, Kirkham FJ, Winstanley PA et al (1991) Intracranial pressure in African children with cerebral malaria. *Lancet* **337**: 573–576.

Newton CR, Peshu N, Kendall B et al (1994) Brain swelling and ischaemia in Kenyans with cerebral malaria. *Archives of Diseases in Childhood* **70**: 281–287.

Pasvol G, Newton CR, Winstanley PA et al (1991) Quinine treatment of severe falciparum malaria in African children: a randomized comparison of three regimens. *American Journal of Tropical Medicine and Hygiene* **45**: 702–713.

Phillips RE, Warrell DA, White NJ et al (1985) Intravenous quinidine for the treatment of severe falciparum malaria. Clinical and pharmacokinetic studies. *New England Journal of Medicine* **312**: 1273–1278.

Poser CM & Roman GC (1991) Cerebral malaria. *Lancet* **337**: 1282.

Pukrittayakamee S, Clemens R, Pramoolsinsap C et al (1992) Polymorphonuclear leukocyte elastase in *Plasmodium falciparum* malaria. *Transactions of the Royal Society of Tropical Medicine and Hygiene* **86**: 598–601.

Pukrittayakamee S, Supanaranond W, Looareesuwan et al (1994) Quinine in severe falciparum malaria: evidence of declining efficacy in Thailand. *Transactions of the Royal Society of Tropical Medicine and Hygiene* **88**: 324–327.

Punyagupta S, Srichaikul T, Nitiyanant P & Petchclai B (1974) Acute pulmonary insufficiency in falciparum malaria: summary of 12 cases with evidence of disseminated intravascular coagulation. *American Journal of Tropical Medicine and Hygiene* **23**: 551–559.

Qinghaosu Antimalaria Coordinating Group (1979) Antimalarial studies on qinghaosu. *Chinese Medical Journal* **92**: 811–816.

Rigdon RH (1944) The pathological lesions in the brain in malaria. *Southern Medical Journal* **37**: 687–694.

Roche RJ, Silamut K, Pukrittayakamee S et al (1990) Quinine induces reversible high-tone hearing loss. *British Journal of Clinical Pharmacology* **29**: 780–782.

Roche G & Helenport J-P (1994) The view of the pharmaceutical industry. *Transactions of the Royal Society of Tropical Medicine and Hygiene* **88 (supplement 1)**: 57–58.

Ross R (1914) Intramuscular injections of quinine. *Journal of Tropical Medicine and Hygiene* **17**: 286–288.

Silamut K & White NJ (1993) Relation of the stage of parasite development in the peripheral blood to prognosis in severe falciparum malaria. *Transactions of the Royal Society of Tropical Medicine and Hygiene* **87**: 436–443.

Silamut K, Molunto P, Ho M et al (1991) Alpha 1-acid glycoprotein (orosomucoid) and plasma protein binding of quinine in falciparum malaria. *British Journal of Clinical Pharmacology* **32**: 311–315.

Strahan JH (1948) Quinine by continuous intravenous drip in the treatment of acute falciparum malaria. *Transactions of the Royal Society of Tropical Medicine and Hygiene* **41**: 669–676.

ter Kuile F, Nosten F, Chongsuphajaisiddhi et al (1992) Absorption of intramuscular phenobarbitone in children with severe falciparum malaria. *European Journal of Clinical Pharmacology* **42**: 107–110.

Waller D, Krishna S, Craddock C et al (1990) The pharmacokinetic properties of intramuscular quinine in Gambian children with severe falciparum malaria. *Transactions of the Royal Society of Tropical Medicine and Hygiene* **84**: 488–491.

Waller D, Crawley J, Nosten F et al (1991) Intracranial pressure in childhood cerebral malaria. *Transactions of the Royal Society of Tropical Medicine and Hygiene* **85**: 362–364.

Warrell DA, Looareesuwan S, Warrell MJ et al (1982) Dexamethasone proves deleterious in cerebral malaria: a double-blind trial in 100 comatose patients. *New England Journal of Medicine* **306**: 313–319.

Warrell DA, Looareesuwan S, Phillips RE et al (1986) Function of the blood-cerebrospinal fluid barrier in human cerebral malaria: rejection of the permeability hypothesis. *American Journal of Tropical Medicine and Hygiene* **35**: 882–889.

White NJ (1991) Lumbar puncture in cerebral malaria. *Lancet* **338**: 640–641.

White NJ (1992) Antimalarial pharmacokinetics and treatment regimens. *British Journal of Clinical Pharmacology* **34**: 1–10.

White NJ (1994) Clinical pharmacokinetics and pharmacodynamics of artemisinin and derivatives. *Transactions of the Royal Society of Tropical Medicine and Hygiene* **88 (supplement 1)**: 41–43.

White NJ & Krishna S (1989) Treatment of malaria: some considerations and limitations of the current methods of assessment. *Transactions of the Royal Society of Tropical Medicine and Hygiene* **83**: 767–777.

White NJ, Looareesuwan S, Warrell DA et al (1982) Quinine pharmacokinetics and toxicity in cerebral and uncomplicated falciparum malaria. *American Journal of Medicine* **73:** 564–572.

White NJ, Looareesuwan S, Warrell DA et al (1983a) Quinine loading dose in cerebral malaria. *American Journal of Tropical Medicine and Hygiene* **32:** 1–5.

White NJ, Looareesuwan S & Warrell DA (1983b) Quinine and quinidine: a comparison of EKG effects during the treatment of malaria. *Journal of Cardiovascular Pharmacology* **5:** 173–175.

White NJ, Watt G, Bergqvist Y & Njelesani EK (1987) Parenteral chloroquine for treating falciparum malaria. *Journal of Infectious Diseases* **155:** 192–201.

White NJ, Miller KD, Churchill FC et al (1988a) Chloroquine treatment of severe malaria in children. Pharmacokinetics, toxicity, and new dosage recommendations. *New England Journal of Medicine* **319:** 1493–1500.

White NJ, Looareesuwan S, Phillips RE et al (1988b) Single dose phenobarbitone prevents convulsions in cerebral malaria. *Lancet* **ii:** 64–66.

White NJ, Krishna S, Waller D et al (1989) Open comparison of intramuscular chloroquine and quinine in children with severe chloroquine-sensitive falciparum malaria. *Lancet* **2:** 1313–1316.

Winstanley PA, Newton CR, Pasvol G et al (1992) Prophylactic phenobarbitone in young children with severe falciparum malaria: pharmacokinetics and clinical effects. *British Journal of Clinical Pharmacology* **33:** 149–154.

Winstanley P, Newton C, Watkins W et al (1993) Towards optimal regimens of parenteral quinine for young African children with cerebral malaria: the importance of unbound quinine concentration. *Transactions of the Royal Society of Tropical Medicine and Hygiene* **87:** 201–206.

Woodruff AW & Dickinson CJ (1968) Use of dexamethasone in cerebral malaria. *British Medical Journal* **3:** 31–32.

World Health Organization (1984) Advances in chemotherapy. *Technical Report Series* Geneva; World Health Organization.

World Health Organization (1986a) Severe and complicated malaria. *Transactions of the Royal Society of Tropical Medicine and Hygiene* **80 (supplement 1):** 1–50.

World Health Organization (1986b) The chemotherapy of malaria. In Bruce-Chwatt LJ (ed.) *WHO Monograph Series* number 27, revised edition. Geneva: World Health Organization.

World Health Organization (1990) Severe and complicated malaria. 2nd edn. *Transactions of the Royal Society of Tropical Medicine and Hygiene* **84 (supplement 2):** 1–65.

World Health Organization (1993) *The role of artemisinin and its derivatives in the current treatment of malaria.* Report of an informal consultation, 27–29 September, Geneva.

Yen LM, Dao LM, Day NPJ et al (1994) The role of quinine in the high mortality of intramuscular quinine tetanus. *Lancet* **344:** 786–787.

7

Malaria prevention and prophylaxis

G. DENNIS SHANKS

The prevention of malaria is controversial due to a lack of easily interpretable information on malaria epidemiology, anti-malarial drugs for prophylaxis and drug resistance. The major issues in prevention are however, clear. Malaria is resurging across wide areas of tropical Africa, Asia and South America. A large and growing number of international travellers visit malarious areas. Health authorities from countries in which there is no endemic malaria transmission are reporting increasing numbers of their citizens who contract malaria in the tropics and then become ill on return home. Most anti-malarial drugs are at least a generation old and are rapidly losing their efficacy as multiple drug resistance evolves and spreads across the globe. Public awareness of exotic diseases is widespread and there is a demand for an easy means of avoiding them without inconvenience to daily routine or travel schedules. Recourse to legal measures if physicians fail to protect patients against rare, lethal diseases or warn them against rare adverse affects is on the increase.

In the face of these developments, it is not surprising that there is no simple consensus on how to best prevent malaria, one of the world's most common lethal infections. Recommended malaria chemoprophylaxis regimens vary widely between Western nations reflecting historical precedents and lack of solid data on which to make informed decisions (Lobel and Keystone, 1994). The spread of chloroquine resistance over the past 30 years has left the world without a cheap, easy-to-use drug which has few side-effects. This chapter will review the current measures used to prevent malaria and attempt to guide physicians through the available data that will allow them to make reasonable decisions to protect both their patients and their practice from undue risk caused by malaria.

The key to prevention is to correctly identify patients at risk and then give them an understandable and practical means of decreasing that risk. Not all travellers to the tropics are at risk for malaria. Most tropical travellers frequent tourist destinations and capital cities where the risk of malaria infection is either very low or non-existent (Steffen and Behrens, 1992). The vast majority of travellers going to South East Asia, South America and North Africa require no chemoprophylaxis for malaria. A careful review of the proposed itinerary including a discussion of the mode of travel and planned lodging is often necessary to determine if the

Baillière's Clinical Infectious Diseases—
Vol. 2, No. 2, July 1995
ISBN 0–7020–1983–6

traveller will be exposed to malaria at all. One should use current public health documents such as the Centers for Disease Control's *Health Information for International Travel* (CDC, 1992), the World Health Organization's *International Travel and Health* (WHO, 1992) or the malaria prophylaxis summary in the *British Medical Journal* (Bradley and Warhurst, 1995) as reasonably authoritative documents. This information, however, is at best incomplete as many areas of the world, especially in tropical Africa and Asia, do not have functional health information systems, realistic diagnostic capacities, or much in the way of health services outside the capital city. A few general rules will assist in identifying the high-risk traveller who requires chemoprophylaxis. SubSaharan Africa, the Amazon basin of South America, tropical forest areas of South East Asia and most islands in Melanesia (New Guinea) have endemic falciparum malaria that is not cured by chloroquine. Malaria risk usually increases as one leaves urban areas and moves farther into the tropical jungle. War, famine and mass public health emergencies with resulting refugee populations often create good conditions for the spread of malaria and other infectious diseases.

Certain types of travellers are at much higher risk of malaria than a commercial traveller who only stays at Western standard hotels in capital cities. Former residents who have immigrated to developed countries and then return to the tropics for family visits are a high-risk group (Lackritz et al, 1991) because they have lost their acquired immunity to malaria and are unaware of the need for preventive measures. People who go into particularly remote areas, such as social scientists doing rural field work or adventure travellers seeking isolated uncivilized areas, are especially at risk. Budget tourists travelling overland ('backpackers') are often unwilling to buy expensive drugs and have little desire to carry mosquito nets in their already full rucksacks. Military units, especially those operating at night and in jungles, have a record of very high malaria attack rates (Black, 1973). A careful history from the prospective traveller is the best means of determining who is actually at high risk for malaria.

People tolerate risk in different and often inconsistent ways. Some individuals have a minimal tolerance for risk of disease or medication side-effects. These people are probably well advised not to visit the tropics. Others seek risks that many would consider unacceptable such as the Special Air Service soldier who parachutes into dense jungle and then travels overland at night to an unknown destination. Between these extremes are most tropical travellers who want to visit the tropics but do not wish to become ill with an unpleasant and potentially lethal disease, especially if the means of prevention are relatively inexpensive and do not interfere with their reason for visiting the tropics. In this situation, one cannot make universally applicable statements. Endeavouring to assess the level of malaria risk of a traveller and applying preventive measures appropriate to this risk and to the traveller's willingness to use such measures, provides a better means of protection than any routine prescription of antimalarial drugs.

MOSQUITO AVOIDANCE MEASURES

Individuals who are not bitten by infected anopheline mosquitoes do not get malaria! Although this is a truism, absolute avoidance of mosquitoes is not possible in most tropical areas. Several means are available, however, to avoid most mosquito bites which, besides reducing the risk of malaria, also protect against other arthropod-borne diseases such as dengue fever and viral encephalitis. Passive avoidance measures such as window screens are well worth the trouble and expense, especially for people who plan to live for extended periods in the tropics. Screens need to be repaired and monitored frequently as mosquitoes are quite adept at discovering alternative means of entry into human habitations. In particular check the area where the wall and ceiling meet as tropical construction sometimes leaves gaps for ventilation which makes window screens useless. Try to keep doors closed and use screened verandas rather than open porches to enjoy the evening air.

The anopheline mosquito responsible for malaria is typically most active in the early evening and during the night. A protected sleeping place is important in the prevention of malaria. Where screens are impractical, bed nets are a good adjunct for the tropical home. Common mistakes with bed nets include a failure to mend holes, allowing one's body to touch the net during the night and not thoroughly tucking in the net's lower edges. Insecticide treatment of bed nets considerably increases their ability to protect the sleeper from mosquitoes and disease (Alonso et al, 1991). Typically the nets are soaked in a permethrin solution every few months. Another adjunctive procedure for bed nets is to use a knock-down spray containing permethrin in the sleeping area about 1 hour before sleeping and after setting the bed net over the bed in order to kill any adult mosquitoes that are already present in the bedroom.

Mosquito repellents are a useful short-term measure to avoid exposure to malaria-infected mosquitoes. Repellents are best applied at about sundown to protect during the early evening prior to sleeping. Most repellents contain N,N-diethyl-m-toluamide (DEET), which is an organic chemical capable of dissolving plastics if put directly on items such as watch crystals, spectacles, sleeping bags etc. Individuals should be warned not to apply DEET directly into eyes, mouth or nose but only on intact skin. Repellents are best used by placing a light application on exposed skin. Wearing long trousers and long sleeves minimizes the exposed skin area. Frequent applications of repellents every few hours is necessary when using liquid formulations especially in very humid areas. There is no particular advantage in obtaining repellents with very high concentrations of DEET (> 50%); it only requires less material to be applied for the same repellent effect. Many volunteer studies and market surveys have indicated that most people prefer cream-based repellent formulations over liquid ones. The controlled-release cream-based repellent (Ultrathon™, Sports Products, 3M, St Paul, MN) provides protection against biting insects (against mosquitoes for up to 12 hours) for longer periods compared to liquid-based repellent formulations (Gupta and Rutledge, 1989). Care should be taken to follow the manufacturer's instructions, as excessive use and absorption of DEET into the body can in rare cases produce seizures (CDC, 1989a).

CHEMOPROPHYLAXIS IN GENERAL

The concept of using anti-malarial drugs to prevent malaria is as old as chemotherapy itself, having been popularized by Robert Koch in the last century. Due to imperfect drugs, adaptable parasites, persistent mosquitoes and human behaviour, malaria chemoprophylaxis has never quite matched its theoretical promise. Despite the spread of drug resistance, it is currently possible to protect the vast majority of travellers who are exposed to malaria from developing the actual disease (Behrens and Roberts, 1994). However, this cannot be done at minimal cost, without the risk of unpleasant side-effects or without the informed cooperation of the traveller. Matching the patient to the appropriate drug for chemoprophylaxis depends not only on pharmacological factors, but also on the epidemiologic issues discussed above. Malaria chemoprophylaxis is indicated for all travellers who are significantly exposed to malaria, as the risk of a rapidly lethal infection with *Plasmodium falciparum* in non-immune individuals is very real (Steffen et al, 1993).

One of the greatest problems in prescribing anti-malarial drugs for prophylaxis is drug regimen compliance by the patient. Many patients whilst carrying anti-malarials do not take them as prescribed. Careful discussion of the actual regimen to be used can partly minimize the problem. Healthy people do not like to take medication especially when they suspect that it might cause unpleasant side-effects. Some budget travellers prefer to believe in local folk-lore to prevent malaria and the use of malaria chemoprophylaxis is discouraged by some travel guidebooks. Military groups which exercise disciplinary sanctions on soldiers not obeying drug administration orders still find that the majority of prophylaxis failures are due to failure of compliance (Sanchez et al, 1993). It is often advantageous to prescribe the simplest regimen possible in order to enhance compliance even though it may not be optimal. Adding a second drug, for example, may include a broader spectrum of coverage, but will reduce compliance. Weekly rather than daily medication will improve compliance. Other travellers insist that it is easier to remember a daily medication and once this habit is part of the morning routine, it is easier to maintain. In any case, it is extremely important for the physician to emphasize that chemoprophylaxis is being prescribed for good medical reasons and should be taken as directed.

Anti-malarial drug resistance is an evolving problem with little hope of a simple solution in sight. The inexorable spread of chloroquine-resistant falciparum malaria has now been followed in close succession by pyrimethamine/sulphadoxine and mefloquine resistance (Kain, 1993). Indeed, in many areas of South East Asia multiple drug resistance has rapidly diminished the efficacy of all anti-malarial drugs (White and Nosten, 1993). The movement of chloroquine-resistance across the African continent from east to west has been rapid and in many areas of East Africa there is also substantial pyrimethamine/sulphadoxine resistance. The first warning of drug failure arises when travellers despite full compliance with chemoprophylaxis develop malaria after returning to a non-endemic country (Raccurt et al, 1991). Vivax malaria is no longer universally sensitive to chloroquine in travellers returning from the Indonesian and Melanesian archipelagoes (Rieckmann et al, 1989; Murphy et al, 1993). The ability of parasites to develop resistance to anti-malarial drugs is so pervasive that it is essential to warn all travellers that the protection provided by anti-malarials is not absolute and that if any fever should develop within several months after return from a tropical country, malaria needs to be excluded.

None of the drugs used in malarial chemoprophylaxis are without side-effects. Although some drugs used for chemoprophylaxis have adverse effects that are well understood, such as haemolysis in glucose-6-phosphate-dehydrogenase (G6PD)-deficient individuals when given prima-quine, most studies describe a range of side-effects that occur unpredictably. Regardless of the actual aetiology, side-effects due to drugs cause travellers to discontinue medication and lead to breakthrough of infection. In a large study of European travellers returning from East Africa, 1–3% of travellers admitted discontinuing chemoprophylaxis due to drug side-effects and 17–35% complained that the drugs had made them ill during travel (Steffen et al, 1993). The 5% background of complaints in those taking no chemoprophylaxis suggests that not all side-effects associated with chemoprophylaxis were due to actual drug effect. It is good medical practice to warn patients beforehand of the commonly associated side-effects of their particular regimen which helps most patients to continue prophylaxis despite minor problems.

Serious adverse effects though rare, do occur. Certain individuals such as airline pilots cannot accept even small risks of side-effects that might jeopardize life should they occur while flying. Mefloquine is not given to air crews for this reason. Several anti-malarial drugs have been abandoned for general use as malaria chemoprophylactic agents because of rare severe adverse effects. These are: amodiaquine, which can cause agranulocytosis (Hatton et al, 1986) and hepatitis (Neftel et al, 1986); pyrimethamine/ sulphadoxine (Fansidar™), which can cause severe cutaneous reactions (Miller et al, 1986); and pyrimethamine/dapsone (Maloprim™), which can cause agranulocytosis (Friman et al, 1983). When drugs are given as chemoprophylaxis the risk/benefit ratio is quite different from when drugs are given for the treatment of serious illnesses (Phillips-Howard and West, 1990).

DIFFICULT GROUPS: CHILDREN, PREGNANT WOMEN, LONG-STAY TRAVELLERS

For ethical or economic reasons, drug companies do not encourage studies seeking to define the tolerance of drugs in children and pregnant women, the two groups most vulnerable to severe infection. Although understandable, this leaves a great gap of information when prescribing chemoprophylaxis for such special groups. Information on drug safety in pregnancy usually comes from limited case reports of women who have become pregnant while on chemoprophylaxis. Where data do not exist, the physician is forced to judge on fragmentary information regarding the drug and the perceived malaria risk of the patient. Most pregnant women should be asked if their travel to an endemic area is necessary, and should also be carefully counselled as to the risks and benefits of the drugs and contracting the disease. Fortunately many anti-malarial drugs have been tested in the treatment of paediatric malaria patients, although this is not so for chemoprophylaxis. Few anti-malarials come in suspensions (chloroquine is an exception) or in tablets that are scored to facilitate accurate dosage in children. Nearly all anti-malarials have a very bitter taste in suspension or when crushed in food.

For long-term travellers, some of the risk assessment for anti-malarial prophylaxis becomes more difficult. Nearly all drugs have the potential to cause problems if taken for long enough. Lack of motivation to continue medication indefinitely causes many expatriates to discontinue prophylaxis. Many believe erroneously that they, like the indigenous people around them, might have gained some degree of immunity and do not require prophylaxis. Long-term expatriates need to be educated about their risk of contracting malaria. Access to medical care, its quality, as well as the difficulty of possible emergency medical evacuation should be considered in the risk/benefit equation for the use of long-term malarial chemoprophylaxis. The physician's task is often one of guiding individuals on a one-to-one basis to an informed decision on how best to prevent malaria infection in their particular situation.

DRUGS CURRENTLY USED FOR CHEMOPROPHYLAXIS

Chloroquine

Chloroquine is a drug that was initially developed in Germany and was the mainstay of treatment and prophylaxis for over a generation after the Second World War. The spread of chloroquine resistance from South East Asia and South America, however, has for the most part made chloroquine redundant for chemoprophylaxis. Chloroquine cannot be relied on to protect travellers to Africa from falciparum malaria (Steffen et al, 1993). For travellers going to the malarious areas of the Middle East, the Caribbean (Haiti) or Central America north of the Panama Canal, weekly chloroquine is still a good prophylactic drug. The identification of chloroquine-resistant vivax malaria in Melanesia (Rieckmann et al, 1989) and in Indonesia (Murphy et al, 1993) has raised questions about using chloroquine even to suppress relapsing malaria. The vast majority of travellers however, require alternative drugs instead of, or in addition to, chloroquine.

Chloroquine is a relatively easy-to-use, cheap drug. The usual adult prophylactic dose is 300 mg of drug base once a week which is the equivalent of the salts, 500 mg chloroquine phosphate or 600 mg chloroquine sulphate. It is important to realize that people substantially greater than 70 kg in weight may need more chloroquine. Liquid paediatric formulations exist which facilitates administration of the paediatric dosage of 5 mg base/kg per week. It is best to start prophylaxis at least 2 weeks prior to travel in order to increase blood concentrations while in the endemic area and to determine if there are any minor side-effects. Medication should be continued for 4 weeks after return to eradicate any residual falciparum infections. Chloroquine can cause sever pruritis in Africans and some individuals suffer dizziness. Chloroquine intoxication is not rare, either accidentally by children or purposefully by adults. Besides the usual treatments of drug overdose to remove excess drug such as activated charcoal (Wilkinson et al, 1993), consider intravenous diazepam to treat the difficult, protracted arrhythmias refractory to conventional therapy which are the most common cause of death (Riou et al, 1988).

Proguanil and its combinations

Proguanil (Paludrine™) is a prodrug of cycloguanil, which is an antifolate compound. Developed by British and Australian scientists during the Second World War, proguanil rapidly lost its ability in the treatment of malaria due to parasite drug resistance. Proguanil has, however, been widely used for many years as a chemoprophylactic drug with an excellent safety and tolerance record; the only commonly reported side-effect is mouth ulcers (Drysdale et al, 1990). Proguanil's action includes causal prophylaxis by killing the liver stages of *P. falciparum*, which, unlike most drugs, prevents blood infection from ever occurring. Resistance to one antifolate compound however, does not necessarily imply resistance to another (Foote et al, 1990). The genetic ability to convert proguanil into cycloguanil efficiently is not universal, and the usefulness of proguanil in some Asian (Edstein et al, 1994a) and African (Watkins et al, 1990) populations has been questioned. Chlorproguanil was originally thought to be longer-acting than proguanil, but weekly dosing did not achieve protection in Kenyan children (Watkins et al, 1987) or in Burundian children receiving either weekly chlorproguanil alone or with chloroquine (Coosemans et al, 1987). Chlorproguanil, like proguanil, probably has to be given daily (Nevill et al, 1994).

A survey of non-immune residents of Dar es Salaam, Tanzania indicated that daily proguanil could be used in combination with weekly chloroquine (McLarty et al, 1984). Several studies in Francophone Africa have popularized either the use of weekly chloroquine (300 mg base/week) combined with daily proguanil (200 mg/day: Gozal et al, 1991) or the use of daily chloroquine (100 mg base/day) and daily proguanil (200 mg/day: Garin et al, 1993). Should one decide to use such combination regimens, it is vital that the patient be very closely instructed so as not to confuse which pills are taken weekly and which are to be administered daily. Despite the attraction of using two relatively safe drugs, a large comparative study of European travellers going to East Africa showed that proguanil combined with chloroquine was decidedly inferior to mefloquine in terms of both efficacy and side-effects (Steffen et al, 1993), as did a study of US Peace Corps volunteers (Lobel et al, 1993). A basic problem when using proguanil and chloroquine is maintaining compliance with this demanding regimen.

Other proguanil combinations have been tried in order to develop anti-folate synergy and to reduce the likelihood of resistance. The Australian Army successfully used daily proguanil combined with 25 mg of daily dapsone during the Vietnam War (Black, 1973), although rare life-threatening haematological complications were seen which prevented this combination ever being used generally. Lower daily doses of dapsone were later used in combination with proguanil in the Thai Army, but poor efficacy was observed against the multiple-drug-resistant falciparum malaria present on the Thai–Cambodian border (Shanks et al, 1992). The good safety record of proguanil prompted the investigation of various proguanil and sulphonamide drug combinations in children on the Thai–Burmese border (Pang et al, 1989; Karwacki et al, 1990). Although promising as an alternative drug in paediatric populations in multiple-drug-resistant areas, testing of proguanil/sulphamethoxazole in semi-immune Thai soldiers on the Cambodian border did not indicate adequate efficacy for general use (Karwacki et al, 1991). Allergic reactions to sulpha drugs as well as the difficulty in giving multiple pills daily did not make these proguanil combinations practical for use outside clinical studies.

Mefloquine

Mefloquine is an anti-malarial drug that was developed by the US Army to prevent chloroquine-resistant falciparum malaria encountered during the Vietnam War. It is related to quinine and halofantrine in that *P. falciparum* parasites tend to develop cross-resistance to all three drugs (Cowman et al, 1994). Early field trials in Thai civilians demonstrated that mefloquine was an excellent chemosuppressive agent (Pearlman et al, 1980). Although mefloquine was originally used in combination with pyrimethamine/sul-phadoxine for treatment (Fansimef™, Hoffmann LaRoche), only meflo-quine on its own has been recommended for chemoprophylaxis. Mefloquine has been successfully used in Africa, particularly in US Peace Corps volunteers and European tourists. The currently recommended adult regimen is 250 mg/week, since alternate week administration results in unacceptable failure rates (Lobel et al, 1991). Mefloquine has a very long half-life. In a recent study, steady state concentrations were achieved after > 10 weeks when given as 250 mg/week to US Marines (Boudreau et al, 1993). Therefore, loading dose regimens are being considered especially in areas with relatively mefloquine-resistant falciparum malaria to prevent breakthrough infections developing soon after initiating prophylaxis. Although the manufacturer places restrictions on the length of time meflo-quine should be used for prophylaxis, the US Peace Corps has successfully used mefloquine for more than 1 year (Lobel et al, 1993). Although there have been reports of mefloquine prevention failures from West Africa (Raccurt et al, 1991), experience from travellers to East Africa supports the use of weekly mefloquine as the best tolerated and most effective regimen (Steffen et al, 1993). Mefloquine is not as yet available in a liquid form and is not recommended by the manufacturer for use in children under 15 kg. Despite this, there is no evidence that it damages the developing fetus (Nosten et al, 1994), and it has been successfully used for the treatment of very young children. Mefloquine does not eliminate relapsing malaria from the liver, so late relapses of vivax and ovale malaria are possible after discontinuation of prophylaxis.

The question of side-effects due to prophylactic mefloquine is a debatable one. Some individuals complain of a vague dysphoria while taking mefloquine; it is unpleasant, undefinable and causes patients to refuse further administration of mefloquine. Serious central nervous system reactions such as seizures and psychotic reactions are much more common when taking treatment courses (estimated incidence 1 in 215) of mefloquine than when taking it for prophylaxis (1 in 13 000: Weinke et al, 1991). Studies of large groups of travellers have consistently shown that mefloquine is well tolerated and is no more of a problem than chloroquine (Steffen et al, 1993; Lobel et al, 1993). However, a randomized controlled trial using chloroquine and mefloquine in US Marines stationed in a non-endemic area showed that men receiving mefloquine had more problems with mind side-effects such as sleep disturbances, vivid dreams and nightmares than those receiving chloroquine (Boudreau et al, 1993). Despite the findings concerning the safety of prophylactic mefloquine, there are indications that neuropsychiatric side-effects are substantially under-reported (Bradley and Warhurst, 1995). Most adverse effects occur after the first few doses of mefloquine. Alternative drugs should be arranged for people who have not tolerated mefloquine previously. Mefloquine should not be given to people taking β-adrenergic antagonists such as propranolol.

Resistance to mefloquine developed rapidly on the Thai–Cambodian border after the widespread use of mefloquine in Thailand (Wongsrichanalai et al, 1992). Multiple-drug-resistance has since spread to the Thai–Burma border (Nosten et al, 1991). Mefloquine prophylaxis failures are not a rare event in soldiers on the Thai–Cambodian border both in semi-immune Thai soldiers (Suriyamongkol et al, 1991) and Dutch Marines (Hopperus-Buma et al, 1993). Mefloquine prophylaxis failures (Shanks et al, 1991) and treatment failures (ter Kuile et al, 1993) are not readily cured with standard regimens of halofantrine. Mefloquine prophylaxis failures often present with few symptoms several weeks after discontinuation of prophylaxis. This makes the accurate diagnosis of a mefloquine prophylaxis failure a difficult task often only confirmed after careful microscopic examination of repeated blood smears. Mefloquine is generally not recommended for areas of known mefloquine-resistance, which currently includes the Cambodian and Burmese borders of Thailand. Doxycycline is usually the recommended prophylaxis for travellers to these areas.

Doxycycline

Tetracyclines are slow blood schizonticides that are used as an adjunct to cure when treating drug-resistant falciparum malaria with quinine. Daily doxycycline (100 mg) was used as a chemoprophylactic against falciparum malaria in adolescent school children on the Thai–Burmese border with good success (Pang et al, 1987). A subsequent trial indicated that daily doxycycline (100 mg) was better than 50 mg daily due to vivax breakthroughs at the lower dosage (Pang et al, 1988). Relapses of vivax malaria commonly occurred after discontinuation of doxycycline prophylaxis. Daily doxycycline has been used successfully by US soldiers deployed on joint field exercises in Thailand since 1987. Suggestions that antibiotic-induced gut flora modification by doxycycline may cause some gastrointestinal problems was dispelled by a blinded, placebo-controlled trial in US soldiers receiving either daily doxycycline or weekly mefloquine (Arthur et al, 1990a). Side-effects were not significantly different between the mefloquine and doxycycline groups (Arthur et al, 1990b). Daily doxycycline should be taken with a meal as it can often cause gastrointestinal upset when taken on an empty stomach. Sun-sensitization is commonly reported when using tetracyclines in the tropics but is usually manageable with sun-block skin creams. A few (1.4%) of the Australian soldiers deployed in Somalia had to discontinue daily doxycycline due to excessive sunburn (unpublished data). Tetracyclines are not given to children < 9 years of age or to pregnant women due to staining of immature teeth and bone. Adult women may develop candida vaginitis when on long-term doxycycline, which often requires discontinuation of the antibiotic.

Daily doxycycline as malaria prophylaxis is highly effective. Thai soldiers on the Cambodian border were able to use daily doxycycline to prevent highly drug-resistant falciparum malaria (Watanasook et al, 1989). The relative failure of doxycycline compared to weekly mefloquine in US soldiers in Somalia was almost certainly due to lack of compliance with the daily regimen (Sanchez et al, 1993). Doxycycline is highly effective in preventing malaria under intense exposure in areas such as Papua New Guinea (Rieckmann et al, 1993). Despite causal prophylaxis found in earlier volunteer studies, this effect is not reliably reproduced in human challenge trials (Shmuklarsky et al, 1994). Even when combined with low-dose primaquine, daily doxycycline cannot provide reliable causal prophylaxis and must be continued for at least 2 weeks after return to a non-endemic area (Shanks et al, 1995). Neither doxycycline nor mefloquine eliminates the hypnozoite stages of relapsing malaria, so one must give primaquine eradication courses (15 or 30 mg of primaquine base daily for 2 weeks) after return to a non-endemic area in order to eliminate relapse potential in heavily exposed people. People should be screened for G6PD prior to administration of primaquine as some ethnic groups deficient in G6PD, particularly those originating from the Mediterranean region or South East Asia, can suffer marked haemolysis when given standard doses of primaquine.

See Table 1 for a summary of the drugs currently used as prophylactics for malaria.

Table 1. Currently used chemoprophylactic agents for malaria.

Drug	Usage	Adult dose	Paediatric dose	Notes
Chloroquine	Only in Middle East, Central America, Caribbean	300 mg base weekly	5 mg/base/kg weekly	Bitter taste Start at least 2 weeks prior to travel Guard against accidental overdoses
Proguanil combinations	Most popular in travellers from Britain and France	200 mg/day	<2 years 50 mg 2–6 years 100 mg 7–10 years 150 mg	Apparently safe in pregnancy Used with chloroquine or antifolate High failure rates in Africa
Mefloquine	Usual recommendation for travellers to Africa	250 mg/week (1 tablet/week)	15–19 kg ¼ tab 20–30 kg ½ tab 31–40 kg ¾ tab	CNS side-effects rare (>1 : 10 000) Many travellers report dysphoria > 10 weeks before steady state
Doxycycline	South East Asia jungles and areas of mefloquine resistance	100 mg/day	Not used in child <9 yrs	Minor GI upset common Best taken with food Daily compliance very important
Primaquine phosphate	To cure vivax malaria, eradication therapy	15–30 mg/day (of drug base) for 2 weeks	0.5 mg/kg/day for 2 weeks No liquid form	Not used in G6PD-deficient people GI upset with higher doses Military uses to prevent relapses

Abbreviations GI, gastrointestinal; G6PD, glucose-6 phosphate dehydrogenase; CNS, central nervous system.

DRUGS THAT MAY BE USED FOR PROPHYLAXIS IN THE FUTURE

Azithromycin

Azithromycin is a new anti-microbial agent of the azalide class which is related to macrolide antibiotics such as erythromycin. Azithromycin has anti-malarial activity and a favourable pharmacokinetic profile which suggests it might be a useful chemoprophylactic agent. Azithromycin has the added advantage over doxycycline in that it can be given to young children and pregnant women. Three out of four volunteers were protected from mosquito challenge when using 500 mg of azithromycin followed by 250 mg daily for 7 days (Kuschner et al, 1994). Further challenge trials are in progress and field trials are planned for 1995. The experience with azithromycin as an anti-malarial is extremely limited and key questions such as dosage regimen and use as a causal prophylactic must still be answered. Azithromycin's expense will remain the major limiting factor in its use.

Halofantrine

Although successfully used for malaria treatment, halofantrine has no role in prophylaxis. Its highly variable bioavailability suggests that any prophylactic use will require a new and better absorbed formulation (Gillespie et al, 1993). Discovery of rare but serious cardiac arrhythmias due to high concentrations of halofantrine do not encourage its use in healthy people seeking to avoid malaria (Nosten et al, 1993). Apparent cross-resistance with mefloquine does not indicate that prophylactic halofantrine will be useful in areas with high levels of mefloquine-resistance (Shanks et al, 1992). One variation of malaria prevention which has been tried is the post-exposure treatment with halofantrine of people who have been heavily exposed to malaria, but who are not yet symptomatic. This specialized use of halofantrine for treatment has been found to be highly successful in French soldiers returning from Africa (Baudon et al, 1990) and in Papua New Guinea copper miners (Shanks et al, 1993).

WR 238605

WR 238605 is a US Army primaquine analogue that was more potent and less toxic than primaquine when tested in the *P. cynomolgi* rhesus (*Macaca mulatta*) monkey test model (Heisey et al, 1988). Mouse and monkey malaria models have demonstrated that WR 238605 has causal prophylactic, radical curative and gametocytocidal activities (Coleman, 1990; Peters et al, 1993). The drug's ability to kill liver stages of relapsing malaria liver parasites in vitro indicates that WR 238605 promises to be not only a replacement for primaquine, but also a prophylactic agent (Fisk et al, 1989). WR 238605 is just entering clinical trials but it is known to be tolerated in uninfected volunteers up to 600 mg as a single oral dose; it has a half-life of approximately 2 weeks (R. Brueckner, unpublished data). Mosquito challenge studies are currently underway at the Walter Reed Army Institute of Research. Should WR 238605 continue to fulfil its early promise as an effective anti-malarial drug, it could prove both a very useful preventive medication for short-term travellers to the tropics and a means of interrupting transmission of malaria through its gametocytocidal effect.

Atovaquone

Atovaquone, originally called BW 566C80, is a hydroxynaphthoquinone that blocks the electron transport chain of mitochondrial respiration (Fry and Pudney, 1992). Currently its clinical uses are to treat pneumocystis pneumonia or toxoplasma encephalitis in human immunodeficiency virus (HIV) infected patients (Falloon et al, 1991; Kovacs et al, 1992). It is also a potent and promising anti-malarial drug (Hudson et al, 1991). In clinical trials in Thailand, it was found that atovaquone had to be combined with either proguanil or doxycycline to stop the development of atovaquone-resistant parasites. In advanced field trials in several tropical countries, a regimen of 3 days of atovaquone combined with proguanil was found to be an extremely successful treatment for multiple-drug-resistant *P. falciparum* (S. Looareesuwan, unpublished data). Prophylactic indications for atovaquone do not yet exist, but atovaquone is being tested in the prophylaxis of pneumocystis pneumonia. Based on animal and in vitro data, it is hoped that atovaquone will be a true causal prophylactic drug (Davies et al, 1993). Atovaquone, like halofantrine, has variable bioavailability and may require reformulation to improve absorption (Rolan et al, 1994).

WR 250417

WR 250417, also known as PS-15, is a new biguanide related to proguanil. It is a prodrug of an earlier compound WR 99210, which was extremely active against multiple-drug-resistant *P. falciparum* but produced significant gastrointestinal intolerance and was subsequently dropped from development. WR 250417 is a very potent compound against multiple-drug-resistant *P. falciparum* infections of Aotus (*Aotus trivirgatus*) monkeys (Canfield et al, 1993). Primates metabolize the prodrug to its active metabolite, WR 99210 (Edstein et al, 1994b). Although not yet in clinical trials, there are good reasons to think that WR 250417 will eventually prove to be a useful treatment drug for pneumocystis pneumonia (Hughes et al, 1993) and falciparum malaria. It is thought that its action is as an antifolate compound. Clinical studies are awaited, but it seems possible that WR 250417 will be used in combination with other drugs such as atovaquone or sulphamethoxazole (Canfield et al, 1993) and may eventually be used like proguanil with which it shares chemical similarities.

See Table 2 for a summary of the drugs that may possibly be used as prophylactics for malaria.

Table 2. Possible future chemoprophylactic agents for malaria.

Drug	Usage	Notes
Azithromycin	Possible substitute for doxycycline	May provide causal prophylaxis in less than daily dosage May be given to children and in pregnancy
Halofantrine	Possible substitute for mefloquine	Mefloquine resistance implies halofantrine cross-resistance Variable bioavailability so may require reformulation Possible cardiotoxicity with lengthened QT interval
WR 238605	Possible substitute for primaquine	Potential single dose eradication therapy to prevent relapses May have a role in causal prophylaxis of malaria May have a role as anti-transmission drug (kills sporozoites)
Atovaquone	Possible causal prophylactic when used with proguanil	Highly efficacious treatment for drug resistant falciparum Under investigation for pneumocystis prophylaxis in HIV patients Very well tolerated but has variable bioavailability
WR 99210/ WR 250417 (a.k.a. PS-15)	Possible causal prophylactic Related to proguanil	250417 is prodrug of 99210 (a very potent antifolate) Human tests showed that 99210 was poorly tolerated 250417 is candidate for new antifolate combinations

STANDBY MEDICATION

When chloroquine resistance was first detected in Africa, one interim measure that was tried to allow the continued use of prophylactic chloroquine was to issue travellers with a single standby treatment dose of pyrimethamine/sulphadoxine (Fansidar™) to take should their prophylaxis fail. This strategy has been superseded by increased drug resistance and can no longer be supported (CDC, 1989b). Most travellers who take standby medication do not have malaria (Fogh et al, 1988; Wetsteyn and de Geus, 1993). Standby medication, be it mefloquine, halofantrine or quinine, has enormous practical problems which cannot be easily resolved without medical expertise. Most travellers are better served by seeking medical advice should they become ill in the tropics in order to identify their actual problem rather than substituting a generic diagnosis of 'malaria'. In the few travellers who genuinely have no access to medical care, treatment doses of mefloquine can be given for emergency use.

CONCLUSIONS

Malaria is a complex parasitic disease with many means to thwart man's efforts to avoid infection. Despite the success of the malaria parasite in developing drug resistance faster than man can produce new anti-malarials, the vast majority of travellers to the tropics can be adequately protected from malaria without great disruption to their activities. Consistent use of mosquito avoidance measures is probably the easiest means of protection, but it is often overlooked by both traveller and physician. The greatest current problem with chemoprophylaxis is not drug resistance, but compliance with drug regimens. The expectation that radically new means of prevention such as malaria vaccines will replace the need for chemoprophylaxis in the near future is unrealistic. Malaria drugs, despite their difficulties, will remain an important means of preventing malaria into the foreseeable future. The physician who manages tropical travellers is well advised to assess travellers' malaria risks carefully, instruct them on mosquito avoidance measures and use either mefloquine or doxycycline chemoprophylaxis in those who are genuinely exposed to drug-resistant falciparum malaria.

SUMMARY

Malaria prevention and chemoprophylaxis is controversial due to the difficulty in obtaining data to resolve questions of compliance, tolerance and efficacy of anti-malarials given to large numbers of healthy people visiting the tropics. Anti-mosquito measures such as screens, repellents and bed nets are simple methods that work well when used consistently. Significant exposure to falciparum malaria requires chemoprophylaxis as the second line of defence. Due to the progression of drug resistance, most travellers to Africa are best managed with weekly mefloquine. Doxycycline is the main alternative for people who do not tolerate mefloquine, who are travelling to areas of mefloquine-resistant malaria or who are capable of complying with a daily medication regimen. Proguanil combinations have a long safety record, but are currently being superseded by mefloquine. There are no simple solutions for difficult groups of travellers such as children and pregnant women. There are potential, new chemoprophylactic agents which offer hope for better drugs in the future. Azithromycin (an antibiotic), halofantrine, (a drug similar to mefloquine), WR 238605 (a primaquine analogue), atovaquone (a hydroxynaphthoquinone), and WR 250417 (a proguanil analogue) are all being examined for possible use as future malaria chemoprophylactic agents. Careful assessment of malaria exposure, instruction on mosquito avoidance measures and informed use of anti-malarial drugs will prevent malaria in most people travelling to the tropics.

REFERENCES

Alonso PL, Lindsay SW, Armstrong JRM et al (1991) The effect of insecticide-treated bed nets on mortality of Gambian children. *Lancet* **337**: 1499–1502.

Arthur JD, Echeverria P, Shanks GD et al (1990a) A comparative study of gastrointestinal infections in United States soldiers receiving doxycycline or mefloquine for malaria prophylaxis. *American Journal of Tropical Medicine and Hygiene* **43**: 608–613.

Arthur JD, Shanks GD, Echeverria P (1990b) Mefloquine prophylaxis. *Lancet* **i**: 972.

Baudon D, Bernard J, Martet G et al (1990) Halofantrine to prevent falciparum malaria on return from malarious areas. *Lancet* **336**: 377.

Behrens RH & Roberts JA (1994) Is travel prophylaxis worth while? Economic appraisal of prophylactic measures against malaria, hepatitis A, and typhoid in travellers. *British Medical Journal* **309**: 918–922.

Black RH (1973) Malaria in the Australian Army in South Vietnam. *Medical Journal of Australia* **1**: 1265–1270.

346 G. D. SHANKS

Boudreau E, Schuster B, Sanchez J et al (1993) Tolerability of prophylactic Lariam regimens. *Tropical Medicine and Parasitology* **44:** 257–265.

Bradley D & Warhurst DC (1995) Malaria prophylaxis: guidelines for travellers from Britain. *British Medical Journal* **310:** 709–714.

Canfield CJ, Milhous WK, Ager AL et al (1993) PS-15: a potent, orally active antimalarial from a new class of folic acid antagonists. *American Journal of Tropical Medicine and Hygiene* **49:** 121–126.

CDC (1989a) Seizures temporally associated with use of DEET insect repellent. *Morbidity and Mortality Weekly Report* **38:** 678–680.

CDC (1989b) Malaria in travelers returning from Kenya: failure of self-treatment with pyrimethamine/sulfadoxine. *Morbidity and Mortality Weekly Report* **38:** 363–364.

CDC (1992) *Health Information for International Travel.* Atlanta: US Public Health Service.

Coleman RE (1990) Sporontocidal activity of the antimalarial WR-238605 against *Plasmodium berghei* Anka in *Anopheles stephensi. American Journal of Tropical Medicine and Hygiene* **42:** 196–205.

Coosemans MH, Barutwanayo M, Onori E et al (1987) Double-blind study to assess the efficacy of chloroproguanil given alone or in combination with chloroquine for malaria chemoprophylaxis in an area with *Plasmodium falciparum* resistance to chloroquine, pyrimethamine and cycloguanil. *Transactions of the Royal Society of Tropical Medicine and Hygiene* **81:** 151–156.

Cowman AF, Galatis D & Thompson JK (1994) Selection for mefloquine resistance in *Plasmodium falciparum* is linked to amplification of the pfmdr 1 gene and cross-resistance to halofantrine and quinine. *Proceedings of the National Academy of Sciences of the USA* **91:** 1143–1147.

Davies CS, Pudney M, Nicholas JC & Sinden RE (1993) The novel hydroxynaphthoquinone 566C80 inhibits the development of liver stages of *Plasmodium berghei* cultured in vitro. *Parasitology* **106:** 1–6.

Drysdale SF, Phillips-Howard PA & Behrens RH (1990) Proguanil, chloroquine, and mouth ulcers. *Lancet* **335:** 164.

Edstein MD, Shanks GD, Teja-Isavadharm P et al (1994a) Genetic polymorphism of oxidative activation of proguanil and dapsone acetylation in Thai soldiers. *British Journal of Clinical Pharmacology* **37:** 67–70.

Edstein MD, Corcoran KD, Shanks GD et al (1994b) Evaluation of WR 250417 (a proguanil analog) for causal prophylactic activity in the *Plasmodium cynomolgi-Macaca mulatta* model. *American Journal of Tropical Medicine and Hygiene* **50:** 181–186.

Falloon J, Kovacs J, Hughes W et al (1991) A preliminary evaluation of 566c80 for the treatment of *Pneumocystis* pneumonia in patients with the acquired immunodeficiency syndrome. *The New England Journal of Medicine* **325:** 1534–1538.

Fisk TL, Millet P, Collins WE & Nguyen-Dinh P (1989) In vitro activity of antimalarial compounds on the exoerythrocytic stages of *Plasmodium cynomolgi* and *P. knowlesi. American Journal of Tropical Medicine and Hygiene* **40:** 235–239.

Fogh S, Schapira A, Bygbjerg IC et al (1988) Malaria chemoprophylaxis in travellers to east Africa: a comparative prospective study of chloroquine plus proguanil with chloroquine plus sulfadoxine-pyrimethamine. *British Medical Journal* **296:** 820–822.

Foote SJ, Galatis D & Cowman AF (1990) Amino acids in the dihydrofolate reductase-thymidylate synthase gene of *Plasmodium falciparum* involved in cycloguanil resistance differ from those involved in pyrimethamine resistance. *Proceedings of the National Academy of Sciences of the USA* **87:** 3014–3017.

Friman G, Nystrom-Rosander C, Jonsell G et al (1983) Agranulocytosis associated with malaria prophylaxis with Maloprim. *British Medical Journal* **286:** 1244–1245.

Fry M & Pudney M (1992) Site of action of the antimalarial hydroxynaphthoquinone, 566C80. *Biochemical Pharmacology* **43:** 1545–1553.

Garin D, Lamarque D, Ringwald P et al (1993) Efficacy of chloroquine-proguanil chemoprophylaxis against malaria in the Central African Republic. *Transactions of the Royal Society of Tropical Medicine and Hygiene* **87:** 304–305.

Gillespie SH, Msaki EP, Ramsay A et al (1993) A new micronized formulation of halofantrine hydrochloride in the treatment of acute *Plasmodium falciparum* malaria. *Transactions of the Royal Society of Tropical Medicine and Hygiene* **87:** 467–469.

Gozal D, Hengy C & Fadat G (1991) Prolonged malaria prophylaxis with chloroquine and proguanil in a nonimmune resident population of an endemic area with a high prevalence of chloroquine resistance. *Antimicrobial Agents and Chemotherapy* **35:** 373–376.

Gupta RK & Rutledge LC (1989) Laboratory evaluation of controlled-release repellent formulations on human volunteers under three climatic regimens. *Journal of the American Mosquito Control Association* **5:** 52–55.

Hatton CSR, Peto TEA, Bunch C et al (1986) Frequency of severe neutropenia associated with amodiaquine prophylaxis against malaria. *Lancet* **1:** 411–413.

Heisey GE, Milhous WK, Hansuklarita P et al (1988) Radical curative properties of WR 238605. *American Society of Tropical Medicine and Hygiene* **39:** 217 (Abstract no. 323).

Hopperus-Buma APCC, Ohrt C, van Thiel PPAM et al (1993) Mefloquine prophylaxis failures in Dutch United Nations Transitional Authority troops in Cambodia. *American Society of Tropical Medicine and Hygiene* **49:** 231 (Abstract no. 269).

Hudson AT, Dickins M, Ginger CD et al (1991) 566C80: a potent broad spectrum anti-infective agent with activity against malaria and opportunistic infections in AIDS patients. *Drugs Experimental Clinical Research* **17:** 427–435.

Hughes WT, Jacobus DP, Canfield C & Killmar J (1993) Anti-*Pneumocystis carinii* activity of PS-15, a new biguanide folate antagonist. *Antimicrobial Agents and Chemotherapy* **37:** 1417–1419.

Kain KC (1993) Antimalarial chemotherapy in the age of drug resistance. *Current Opinion in Infectious Diseases* **6:** 803–811.

Karwacki JJ, Shanks GD, Limsomwong N & Singharaj P (1990) Proguanil-sulphonamide for malaria prophylaxis. *Transactions of the Royal Society of Tropical Medicine and Hygiene* **84:** 55–57.

Karwacki JJ, Shanks GD, Suriyamongkol V et al (1991) Proguanil/sulfamethoxazole malaria chemoprophylaxis on the Thai-Cambodian border. *Southeast Asian Journal of Tropical Medicine and Public Health* **22:** 77–80.

Kovacs JA et al (1992) Efficacy of atovaquone in treatment of toxoplasmosis in patients with AIDS. *Lancet* **340:** 637–638.

Kuschner RA, Heppner DG, Anderson SL et al (1994) Azithromycin prophylaxis against a chloroquine-resistant strain of *Plasmodium falciparum*. *Lancet* **343:** 1396–1397.

ter Kuile FO, Dolan G, Nosten F et al (1993) Halofantrine versus mefloquine in treatment of multidrug-resistant falciparum malaria. *Lancet* **341:** 1044–1049.

Lackritz EM, Lobel HO, Howell BJ et al (1991) Imported *Plasmodium falciparum* malaria in American travelers to Africa. *Journal of the American Medical Association* **265:** 383–385.

Lobel HO & Keystone JS (1994) Confusion on malaria chemoprophylaxis. *Lancet* **343:** 183.

Lobel HO, Bernard KW, Williams SL et al (1991) Effectiveness and tolerance of long-term malaria prophylaxis with mefloquine. *Journal of the American Medical Association* **265:** 361–364.

Lobel HO, Miani M, Eng T et al (1993) Long-term malaria prophylaxis with weekly mefloquine. *Lancet* **341:** 848–851.

McLarty DG, Jaatinen M, Murru M et al (1984) Chemoprophylaxis of malaria in non-immune residents in Dar es Salaam, Tanzania. *Lancet* **i:** 656–659.

Miller KD, Lobel HO, Satriale RF et al (1986) Severe cutaneous reaction among American travelers using pyrimethamine-sulfadoxine for malaria prophylaxis. *American Journal of Tropical Medicine and Hygiene* **35:** 451–458.

Murphy GS, Basri H, Purnomo et al (1993) Vivax malaria resistant to treatment and prophylaxis with chloroquine. *Lancet* **341:** 96–100.

Neftel KA, Woodtly W, Schmid M et al (1986) Amodiaquine induced agranulocytosis and liver damage. *British Medical Journal* **292:** 721–723.

Nevill CG, Lury JD, Mosobo MK et al (1994) Daily chlorproguanil is an effective alternative to daily proguanil in the prevention of *Plasmodium falciparum* malaria in Kenya. *Transactions of the Royal Society of Tropical Medicine and Hygiene* **88:** 319–320.

Nosten F, ter Kuile F, Chongsuphajaisiddhi T et al (1991) Mefloquine-resistant falciparum malaria on the Thai–Burmese border. *Lancet* **337:** 1140–1143.

Nosten F, ter Kuile FO, Luxemburger C et al (1993) Cardiac effects of antimalarial treatment with halofantrine. *Lancet* **341:** 1054–1056.

Nosten F, ter Kuile F, Maelankiri L et al (1994) Mefloquine prophylaxis prevents malaria during pregnancy: a double-blind, placebo-controlled study. *Journal of Infectious Diseases* **169:** 595–603.

Pang LW, Boudreau EF, Limsomwong N & Singharaj P (1987) Doxycycline prophylaxis for falciparum malaria. *Lancet* **i:** 1161–1164.

Pang L, Limsomwong N & Singharaj P (1988) Prophylactic treatment of vivax and falciparum malaria with low-dose doxycycline. *Journal of Infectious Diseases* **158:** 1124–1127.

Pang LW, Limsomwong N, Singharaj P & Canfield CJ (1989) Malaria prophylaxis with proguanil and sulfisoxazole in children living in a malaria endemic area. *Bulletin of the World Health Organisation* **67**: 51–58.

Pearlman EJ, Doberstyn EB, Sudsok S et al (1980) Chemosuppressive field trials in Thailand IV. The suppression of P. falciparum and P. vivax parasitemias by mefloquine. *American Journal of Tropical Medicine and Hygiene* **29**: 1131–1137.

Peters W, Robinson BL & Milhous WK (1993) The chemotherapy of rodent malaria LI. Studies on a new 8-aminoquinoline, WR 238605. *Annals of Tropical Medicine and Parasitology* **87**: 547–552.

Phillips-Howard PA & West LJ (1990) Serious adverse drug reactions to pyrimethamine-sulphadoxine, pyrimethamine-dapsone and to amodiaquine in Britain. *Journal of the Royal Society of Medicine* **83**: 82–85.

Raccurt CP, Dumestre-Toulet V, Abraham E et al (1991) Failure of falciparum malaria prophylaxis by mefloquine in travelers from West Africa. *American Journal of Tropical Medicine and Hygiene* **45**: 319–324.

Rieckmann KH, Davis DR & Hutton DC (1989) *Plasmodium vivax* resistance to chloroquine? *Lancet* **ii**: 1183–1184.

Rieckmann KH, Yeo AET, Davis DR et al (1993) Recent military experience with malaria chemoprophylaxis. *Medical Journal of Australia* **158**: 466–449.

Riou B, Barriot P, Rimailho A & Baud FJ (1988) Treatment of severe chloroquine poisoning. *New England Journal of Medicine* **318**: 1–6.

Rolan PE, Mercer AJ, Weatherley BC et al (1994) Examination of some factors responsible for a food-induced increase in absorption of atovaquone. *British Journal Clinical Pharmacology* **37**: 13–20.

Sanchez JL, DeFraites RF, Sharp TW & Hanson RK (1993) Mefloquine or doxycycline prophylaxis in US troops in Somalia. *Lancet* **341**: 1021–1022.

Shanks GD, Watt G, Edstein MD et al (1991) Halofantrine for the treatment of mefloquine chemoprophylaxis failures in *Plasmodium falciparum* infections. *American Journal of Tropical Medicine and Hygiene* **45**: 488–491.

Shanks GD, Edstein MD, Suriyamongkol V et al (1992) Malaria chemoprophylaxis using proguanil/dapsone combinations on the Thai–Cambodian border. *American Journal of Tropical Medicine and Hygiene* **46**: 643–648.

Shanks GD, Edstein MD, Kereu RK et al (1993) Postexposure administration of halofantrine for the prevention of malaria. *Clinical Infectious Diseases* **17**: 628–631.

Shanks GD, Barnett A, Edstein MD & Rieckmann KH (1995) Effectiveness of doxycycline combined with primaquine for malaria prophylaxis. *Medical Journal of Australia* **162**: 306–310.

Shmuklarsky MJ, Boudreau EF, Pang LW et al (1994) Failure of doxycycline as a causal prophylactic agent against *Plasmodium falciparum* malaria in healthy nonimmune volunteers. *Annals of Internal Medicine* **120**: 294–299.

Steffen R & Behrens RH (1992) Travellers' malaria. *Parasitology Today* **8**: 61–66.

Steffen R, Fuchs E, Schildknecht J et al (1993) Mefloquine compared with other malaria chemoprophylactic regimens in tourists visiting East Africa. *Lancet* **341**: 1299–1303.

Suriyamongkol V, Timsaad S & Shanks GD (1991) Mefloquine chemoprophylaxis of soldiers on the Thai–Cambodian border. *Southeast Asian Journal of Tropical Medicine and Public Health* **22**: 515–518.

Watanasook C, Singharaj P, Suriyamongkol V et al (1989) Malaria prophylaxis with doxycycline in soldiers deployed to the Thai–Kampuchean border. *Southeast Asian Journal of Tropical Medicine and Public Health* **20**: 61–64.

Watkins WM, Oloo AJ, Gilles HM et al (1987) Inadequacy of chloroproguanil 20 mg per week as chemoprophylaxis for falciparum malaria in Kenya. *Lancet* **i**: 125–128.

Watkins WM, Mberu EK, Nevill CG et al (1990) Variability in the metabolism of proguanil to the active metabolite cycloguanil in healthy Kenyan adults. *Transactions of the Royal Society of Tropical Medicine and Hygiene* **84**: 492–495.

Weinke T, Trautmann M, Held T et al (1991) Neuropsychiatric side effects after the use of mefloquine. *American Journal of Tropical Medicine and Hygiene* **45**: 86–91.

Wetsteyn JCFM & de Geus A (1993) Comparison of three regimens for malaria prophylaxis in travellers to east, central and southern Africa. *British Medical Journal* **307**: 1041–1043.

White NJ & Nosten F (1993) Advances in chemotherapy and prophylaxis of malaria. *Current Opinion in Infectious Diseases* **6**: 323–330.

Wilkinson R, Mahatane J, Wade P & Pasvol G (1993) Chloroquine poisoning. *British Medical Journal* **307:** 504.

Wongsrichanalai C, Webster HK, Wimonwattrawatee T et al (1992) Emergence of multidrug-resistant *Plasmodium falciparum* in Thailand: in vitro tracking. *American Journal of Tropical Medicine and Hygiene* **47:** 112–116.

World Health Organization (1992) *International Travel and Health* Geneva: World Health Organization.

8

The contribution of molecular biology to our understanding of malaria

ROSS L. COPPEL

The last 20 years have seen major advances in our molecular under-standing of malaria parasites, particularly *Plasmodium falciparum*. Three key developments have enabled these advances. The first was the in vitro cultivation system which allowed continuous culture of asexual stages of *P. falciparum*, providing parasites for biochemical studies and for extrac-tion of DNA and RNA. The requirements of growing parasites for human red blood cells and human serum in the early culture systems imposed limitations of scale on the amount of parasite material that could be pro-duced and on the therapeutic uses of such material. This in turn has influenced the type of experiments performed, so that for example, there are few reported studies of protein sequence determination by direct sequencing of proteins. Culture-derived material is considered unsuitable for use in vaccines because of the risk of spread of infectious agents present in the blood or serum used, and of induction of autoimmunity. Further, the number of people who would benefit from the use of a malaria vaccine are so large that mass methods of production and delivery of a vaccine are required. A considerable number of studies have focused therefore on production of recombinant proteins and peptides in various host–vector combinations, or the use of live bacterial or viral vaccine delivery systems.

The second important development in malaria was the generation of panels of monoclonal antibodies for characterization of specific proteins. The addition of particular monoclonals to culture inhibited the growth of parasites suggesting that the corresponding parasite antigens may be useful components of a subunit vaccine.

Third, and most significantly, was the use of the set of technologies collectively known as recombinant DNA, which overcame limitations of the amount of parasite material available for study. Gene libraries derived from either cDNA or genomic DNA and, subsequently, gene sequences derived by use of the polymerase chain reaction (PCR), became the common tools of study. Molecular studies have focused on *P. falciparum*, the causative agent of the most serious form of human malaria, and these studies will form the main substance of this chapter with occasional mention of some of the other malarial parasites.

Baillière's Clinical Infectious Diseases—
Vol. 2, No. 2, July 1995
ISBN 0–7020–1983–6

351

BASIC MOLECULAR BIOLOGY OF *PLASMODIA*

During its life cycle, the DNA content of the parasite nucleus varies. The asexual blood stage of the parasite is haploid, i.e. there is only one copy of each chromosome. Gamete fusion in the mosquito results in the formation of the diploid zygote, and a process of meiotic division takes place. This sexual stage of the life cycle allows gametes of different parasites to exchange genetic material, and modify the antigenic repertoire of the parasite. The process of division eventually leads to formation of a sporozoite which is again haploid (Weber, 1988, 1989).

The genome of *P. falciparum* is remarkably AT rich with an average GC content of 18%. By way of comparison the GC content of *Escherichia coli* nuclear DNA is 50%, of *Mycobacterium tuberculosis* 67% and of human 37%. The unusual base composition of *P. falciparum* DNA makes large genomic fragments unstable when cloned in *E. coli* hosts, and deletions and re-arrangements of clones in genomic libraries have bedevilled much of the molecular work undertaken on this organism. Indeed it has proved impossible so far to construct a conventional genomic library of *P. falciparum* in *E. coli* that covers the entire genome. The development of the PCR and direct sequencing of PCR products has helped greatly in overcoming this technical problem by removing the requirement for a cloning step in a bacterial host.

The AT content of other human and simian malarias is much lower than 81% (in the range of 70%), whereas the AT content of murine and avian malarias is of a similar level to that of *P. falciparum*. On this basis it has been suggested that *P. falciparum* is most closely related to these latter groups of malaria and may have reached man via some form of lateral transfer, relatively late in evolutionary time. Although this might, at first sight, help explain the severe pathology caused by *P. falciparum* infection, the idea that parasites evolve towards minimal virulence with time is no longer considered valid. Recent work clearly demonstrates that long established parasites may be lethal for their hosts (Anderson and May, 1991).

Sequence analysis of the small subunit ribosomal genes (Waters, 1994) also suggests that *P. falciparum* is most closely related to the avian malarias *P. gallinaceum* and *P. lophurae*. In contrast, *P. vivax* is most similar to the monkey malarias of South East Asia and may have first appeared in that geographical area. The quartan malaria, *P. malariae*, has a distinct lineage that clusters neither with avian nor simian malarias, which may suggest an ancient and distinct origin for this organism.

GENES AND ANTIGENS OF MALARIA

Large numbers of *P. falciparum* genes, encoding both antigens and housekeeping proteins, have been cloned. A common approach has been the screening of expression libraries using both patient and experimentally raised antisera. Indeed, much of the technology of expression screening, which is now widespread in all areas of molecular biology, was pioneered in the malaria field. Once a clone was identified, it was used to produce an antiserum, either by affinity purification on the expressing clone or by immunization of laboratory animals. This antiserum would then be used in a number of assays such as immunoblots, immunofluorescence, immunoprecipitation and immunoelectron microscopy to provide data about the protein encoded by the gene, such as molecular mass, localization and stage specificity. Space limitations prevent a comprehensive discussion of the many known gene sequences, but I have provided a listing of many of these genes, their corresponding proteins and abbreviations used in the text in Table 1. Further details of malaria antigen structure and immunogenicity may be found in recent reviews (Howard and Pasloske, 1993; Coppel et al, 1994). The nomenclature of these genes is confused, as happens in most rapidly developing fields, and those interested in the latest information can access the World Health Organization Malaria Database on the Internet. This repository may be reached by anonymous ftp at wehi1.wehi.edu.au or by the world wide web at www.wehi.edu.au.

A surprising feature of many malarial proteins, and of *P. falciparum*, proteins in particular, is the presence in the sequence of arrays of tandemly repeated peptide sequences. Although repetitive proteins have been described in several parasitic organisms such as trypanosomes, *Leishmania* and *Giardia*, there appears to be a greater number of such antigens in *P. falciparum*. The repeat regions may account for an extensive region of the protein and, depending on the particular antigen, the repeat array may be composed of exact copies or be highly degenerate in sequence. The repeats are often charged and cause proteins to migrate anomalously slowly in sodium dodecyl sulphate/polyacrylamide gels. Accordingly, a large number of apparently high molecular mass proteins expressed by *P. falciparum*, e.g. proteins 11–1 and Ag332, have apparent molecular masses of greater than 1000 kDa. An important immunological consequence of these repeat arrays is that they tend to be immunodominant, often focusing the antibody response on particular regions of the protein. Genetic processes can alter the repeat sequences relatively rapidly, allowing major antigenic alterations and a means of escaping immune damage.

Many *P. falciparum* antigens occur in antigenically distinct forms of the same protein expressed by distinct parasite isolates. The repertoire for some of these variant antigens is large and is estimated to be between 50 and 100 for the S-antigens and apical membrane antigen-1 (AMA-1). A different form of variation is demonstrated by the PfEMP-1 protein of *P. falciparum* which undergoes true antigenic variation such that progeny of a clonal parasite line can express a new PfEMP-1 serotype, serologically distinct from the parental cloned line (Roberts et al, 1993). At the time of writing, the first reports are appearing that the elusive genes encoding this particularly important family of proteins had been cloned. Distinct proteins are expressed in each of the life cycle stages and some of these are listed in Table 1. Also, there are numerous proteins expressed in all stages of the life cycle, resulting in an estimated repertoire of 5000–10 000 proteins in *P. falciparum*.

Table 1. Features of proteins of *P. falciparum* for which the gene sequence is known.

Protein	Full name and alternative nomenclature	Molecular mass (kDa)	Location	Comments
A. Sporozoite and exoerythrocytic stage antigens				
CSP-1*	Circumsporozoite protein-1	60	Sporozoite surface	GPI anchored. Motif that binds to hepatocyte Conserved B cell epitope in central repeat and variable T cell epitope
SSP-2*	Sporozoite surface protein-2; TRAP	75	Sporozoite surface	Extensive repeats. Peptides from this protein bind to a protective HLA B27 haplotype in Nigerians
LSA-1	Liver specific antigen 1	140	Exoerythrocytic form	
STARP	Sporozoite threonine and asparagine rich protein	78	Sporozoite surface, liver stage and early asexual stages	2 repeat regions of 45 and 10 residues. No classical membrane anchor
B. Asexual stage antigens				
(i) Predominantly merozoite location				
MSP-1*	Merozoite surface antigen-1; MSA-1, PMMSA, MSPP, p190, gp185, gp195, PSA	185–220	Merozoite surface	Dimorphic forms undergo recombination to generate recombinant variants. Extensive antigenic polymorphism
MSP-2*	Merozoite surface antigen-2; MSA-2, QF122, GYMMSA, gp56	35–56	Merozoite surface	Extensive repetitive sequences. Extensive antigenic polymorphism
AMA-1*	Apical membrane antigen-1; Pf83	82/66	Apical region; neck of rhoptry and merozoite surface	Extensive antigenic polymorphism. Processed to a smaller protein
EBA-175	Erythrocyte binding antigen of 175 kDa; SABP	175	Micronemes and merozoite surface	Membrane anchored, then cleaved for release. Region that binds to glycophorin A has been mapped
SPAM	Secreted protein associated with merozoites, MSP-3	46–75	Parasitophorous vacuole and non-covalently attached to merozoite surface	Extensive heptad based α helical structure. Processed to a smaller mature protein. Extensive antigenic polymorphism.
RhopH3		103–110	Rhoptry body	Binds to RBC surface during invasion. Forms a complex with two other rhoptry proteins
RAP-1*	Rhoptry associated protein-1	80/65	Rhoptries	Forms a molecular complex with RAP-2
RAP-2*	Rhoptry associated protein-2, pf41	43/40	Rhoptries	Forms a molecular complex with RAP-1
Ag512		55	Rhoptries	GPI-anchored protein
(ii) Predominantly mature forms				
MESA	Mature-parasite-infected surface antigen-2; PfEMP-2	250–285	RBC internal surface	Binds to RBC protein 4.1. Extensive repetitive sequences
KAHRP	Knob associated histidine rich protein; HRP-I, KP	80–105	RBC internal surface at knobs	Binds to RBC spectrin. Extensive repetitive sequences

		Size (kDa)	Location	Comments
Ag332		1200	RBC internal surface	Extensive repetitive sequences
41–2		29	RBC internal surface	
GBP	Glycophorin binding protein; Pf120, 96R	96–130	RBC cytoplasm	Binding to glycophorin unlikely to be physiologically relevant. Extensive repetitive sequences
GBP H	Glycophorin binding protein homologue	130	RBC cytoplasm	Extensive degenerate repetitive sequences
FIRA	Falciparum interspersed repeat antigen	>300	RBC cytoplasm	Extensive repetitive sequences
HRP-II	Histidine rich protein-II	60–100	RBC membrane and reported to be secreted	
HRP-III		29–50	Parasite cytoplasm	Extensive repetitive sequences
S-antigen		45–220	Parasitophorous vacuole of schizonts	Extensive repetitive sequences. Extensive antigenic polymorphism
SERA	Serine rich antigen; SERP, p 113, p126, Pf 140	113–140	Parasitophorous vacuole of schizonts	Sequence homologies suggest that SERA may be a protease
SERP H	Serine rich protein homologue	130	Parasitophorous vacuole of schizonts	Extensive repetitive sequences
GLURP	Glutamate rich protein	145	Parasitophorous vacuole of schizonts	Extensive repetitive sequences
ABRA	Acidic basic repeat antigen; p101	110	Parasitophorous vacuole of schizonts	Extensive repetitive sequences
CARP	Clustered asparagine rich protein	36?	Parasite cytoplasm	
R45		160	Parasite cytoplasm of trophozoites	Homology with serine protein kinases
ORA	Octapeptide repeat antigen	140?	Parasitophorous vacuole of trophozoites and schizonts	Extensive repetitive sequences

(iii) Present in most or all stages

RESA	Ring-infected erythrocyte surface antigen; Pf155	155	Dense granules and RBC internal surface in ring-infected RBC	Binds to RBC spectrin. Domain homologous to chaperonins. Extensive repetitive sequences
Exp-1	Exported protein-1, CRA, QF116	23	Vesicles in RBC cytoplasm	Also expressed in liver stages
ARP	Asparagine rich protein	220, 160	Parasite cytoplasm	Extensive repetitive sequences
hsp70-1	Heat shock protein-1, p75	75	Parasite cytoplasm	
hsp70-2	Heat shock protein-2, Pfgrp	70–72	Parasite cytoplasm	Sequence suggests it is a homologue of a chaperonin
Aldolase		41	Parasite cytoplasm	

C. *Sexual stage antigens*

Pfs230*		230	Surface	Expressed in gametocytes and gametes. Target of transmission blocking immunity
Pfs25*		25	Surface	Expressed in ookinetes. Contains several EGF like domains. Target of transmission blocking immunity
Pfs16		16	Parasitophorous vacuole	Expressed in gametes and sporozoites
11.1		>1000	Granules in parasite	Expressed in gametocytes. Deleted from strains that cannot make gametocytes

Those antigens with asterisks are some of those undergoing extensive evaluation as components of a malaria vaccine.

THE CIRCUMSPOROZOITE PROTEIN

Perhaps most data has been gathered about the circumsporozoite protein (CSP-1), an approximately 60 kDa protein located on the surface of developing and mature sporozoites, and present in liver cells containing developing exoerythrocytic forms. The sequence of the gene encoding CSP-1 has been determined in several malaria species and for many distinct isolates of *P. falciparum*. All share a common overall structure. The sequences encode an amino-terminal hydrophobic region that has features consistent with a signal sequence, and a second hydrophobic region at the carboxy terminus is responsible for anchoring the CSP-1 in the sporozoite surface membrane. The central domain of CSP-1 is composed of an extensive array of tandemly repeated short sequences. For the *P. falciparum* CSP-1 of the 7G8 cloned line this region is composed of 37 copies of NANP interspersed with four copies of NVDP. Different isolates have somewhat different numbers of these two tetrapeptides but their presence is conserved throughout all *P. falciparum* isolates. Other malarial species have central repeat domains of differing sequence, e.g. *P. vivax* has a total of 19 copies of two nonapeptides, DRADGQPAG and DRAAGQPAG (Kemp et al, 1987). This repeat region is the target of antibodies that in high enough titre can prevent sporozoites invading liver cells.

Comparison of the complete sequences of the *P. falciparum* and *P. knowlesi* circumsporozoite (CS) proteins show only two short regions of homology. The second region (residues TEWSPCS<u>VTCG</u>NG in *P. falciparum*) is the most highly conserved region among CS proteins of different species, and a related sequence is present in the complement protein, properdin, in thrombospondin and in von Willebrand's factor. Many of the proteins that bear the VTCG related sequence bind to sulphated glyco-conjugates such as dextran sulphate, heparin and fucoidan. Recombinant CS protein from several species binds to sulphated glycoconjugates either coated on sepharose or present on cell surfaces (Pancake et al, 1992). Sporozoite binding to hepatocytes can be inhibited by synthetic peptides from region II or by fucoidan or heparin.

Immune responses to the CS protein may block sporozoite invasion or the development of exoerythrocytic forms of the parasite. The route to immunity may be antibody-based or by the induction of cytotoxic T cells. Considerable ingenuity has been expended in developing immunogenic forms of the CS protein, and virtually every delivery system imaginable has been used. Subunit formulations have included recombinant protein made in *E. coli* and yeast, CS protein fragments fused to various other molecules, synthetic peptides, proteosomes and multiple antigenic peptide arrays with a cornucopia of adjuvant formulations. Live delivery systems have included vaccinia virus, avirulent *Salmonella* and plant virus particles. Most recently, direct injection of DNA molecules has been investigated (Sedegah et al, 1994). No method has proved capable of inducing sufficiently high levels of effective immunity in individuals of diverse genetic backgrounds. A solution to the problem of immunogenicity remains the major challenge to successful vaccine production.

CHROMOSOMAL ORGANIZATION OF MALARIA PARASITES

Malaria parasites are difficult organisms to work with genetically. They have a complex life cycle which limits the feasibility of performing genetic cross experiments. The chromosomes do not condense during meiosis, so that conventional cytogenetics is not possible. Finally, there is no readily available transformation system, which limits the type of experiments that can be performed. The only available genetic tools are libraries of clones and characterized genes and the technique of pulsed field gradient electrophoresis (PFGE). PFGE is a technique for separating very large DNA molecules, in the size range of 100×10^3 base-pairs (kb) to several megabases (Mb), on agarose gels. These separated fragments are then visualized by various means (Schwartz and Cantor, 1984). Chromosomes migrate as discrete bands and PFGE allowed the recognition of malaria chromosomes for the first time. Malarial parasites contain 14 chromosomes which total approximately 30 Mb of genetic information (Foote and Kemp, 1989). By comparison, the size of the human genome is about 3000 Mb and the size of the *E. coli* genome is about 4 Mb. In *P. falciparum*, chromosomes vary in size from between about 630 kb to 3 Mb and surprisingly, an individual chromosome may differ in size by several hundred kilobases in different isolates of the parasite. This marked size variation of chromosomes is found both in parasites cultured in the laboratory and in parasites isolated from patients. There are no sex chromosomes, and a cloned line of malaria can give rise to both male and female gametocytes (Foote and Kemp, 1989). There are other DNA molecules within the malaria genome that are not part of the 14 chromosomes, including a 5.8 kb element and a 30 kb circular molecule. The 5.8 kb element appears to be related to mitochondrial DNA from other species, whereas the 30 kb circle appears most closely related to chloroplast elements found in plants (Gardner et al, 1993). The analysis of nuclear-encoded genes suggests that *Plasmodium* as a genus has a common ancestry with dinoflagellates (Waters, 1994).

The structure of malarial chromosomes is typical of other eukaryotes (Triglia et al, 1992; Lanzer et al, 1994). The ends of the chromosomes are capped by telomeric structures composed of heptanucleotide repeats. In the subtelomeric region there is a complex series of repeats including many copies of a 21 base-pair (bp) sequence that has been used in DNA based diagnostic tests for parasitaemia. The dramatic size polymorphisms of individual chromosomes is due to differences in the length of the subtelomeric region of the chromosome. The 21 bp repeats can vary greatly in number or be completely absent. The subtelomeric region of the chromosome appears to be a rather unstable structure. During mitotic growth of the parasite in culture, chromosomes within individual parasites occasionally undergo a process of breakage, in or near this subtelomeric region, in which part of the chromosome is lost. This can occasionally lead to the loss of a structural gene, often coding for proteins that interact with the red blood cell membrane skeleton (Scherf and Mattei, 1992). Many of these proteins are not required for growth in in vitro culture, and the parasite can survive.

Similar gene loss is not found in isolates taken and analyzed directly from the wild, suggesting that these proteins are essential for parasite survival in the circulation.

The placement of many individual *P. falciparum* genes on the various chromosomes is known and a reasonably comprehensive genomic map is being established (Figure 1). Early data suggests that many of the antigen genes are located near the ends of chromosomes, whereas housekeeping genes appear to cluster centrally. The reason for this arrangement is not known and it may be an artefact of the incomplete process of gene assignment. However, it may be that as many of these genes contain repetitive segments that differ in size in different isolates of parasites, the location in the unstable subtelomeric region may facilitate the process of alteration of antigen repeat sequence and repeat numbers.

Many of the antigens that are important vaccine candidates have been located on the chromosome maps. Merozoite surface protein-1 (MSP-1) maps to chromosome 1, MSP-2 maps to chromosome 2, AMA-1 maps to chromosome 11 and S antigen maps to chromosome 10. Although each antigen exists as a single copy in a particular parasite, within the total population of different parasite strains, each of these antigens is present in many different allelic forms. If a mosquito should feed on more than one infected individual or on an individual infected with multiple strains, the gametocytes in the blood meal can cross-fertilize each other giving rise to new combinations of these antigens in the parasites that develop. Such 'recombinant' parasites will express combinations of the antigens that are different from either parental form and may be able to evade the host immune response more easily.

The Wellcome Trust has funded a consortium of laboratories in a genome project for malaria, the ultimate aim of which is to provide the complete sequence of the *P. falciparum* genome. In its initial stages, the project plans to produce a complete physical map of the genome and provide a library of yeast artificial chromosome (YAC) clones containing large fragments of malaria chromosomes. These YAC clones will be assembled into contiguous arrangements that encompass the entire 14 chromosomes (Triglia et al, 1992). Such a map will provide a basis for further studies on characterization of various genetic loci.

GENETIC MECHANISMS OF DRUG RESISTANCE

The mainstay of malaria control by physicians has been the use of specific drugs for both prophylaxis and therapy. The emergence of multiple-drug-resistant strains of *P. falciparum* worldwide has been both rapid and devastating in scope over the past three decades, and strains resistant to one or several of almost all the commonly used anti-malarial drugs except doxycycline, have been described. The description of *P. vivax* strains resistant to chloroquine has been an unwelcome recent development (Murphy et al, 1993). A clear understanding of resistance mechanisms is essential to the design of countermeasures and new regimens of administration. We

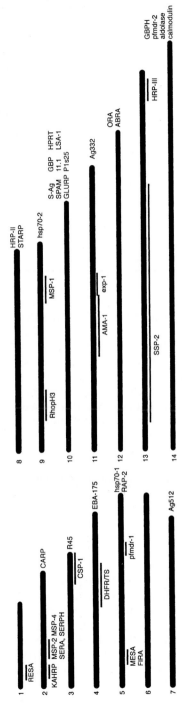

Figure 1. Schematic showing localization of some important *P. falciparum* genes on the 14 chromosomes. In the current state of the map genes are localized to a restriction enzyme fragment that is larger than the total length of the gene. Genes that have been mapped to a chromosome but not to a specific fragment are listed to the right of the corresponding chromosome. Abbreviations are the same as used in Table 1.

understand in detail the mechanisms of resistance to antifolate drugs such as pyrimethamine and cycloguanil, however resistance to chloroquine and other quinoline-type drugs is not as well understood (Table 2). More detailed coverage of the subject of drug resistance can be found in recent reviews by Cowman and Foote (1990) and Foote and Cowman (1994).

Table 2. Putative mechanisms of drug resistance in *P. falciparum* against commonly used chemotherapeutics.

Drug	Target enzyme(s)	Suggested mechanism of resistance
Sulphadoxine	DHPS	Mutation in the target enzyme
Dapsone	DHPS	Mutation in the target enzyme
Pyrimethamine	DHFR	Mutation in the target enzyme
Cycloguanil	DHFR	Mutation in the target enzyme
Chloroquine	Pfmdr1 and others	Multigenic mechanism. Mutation in *pfmdr1* is partly responsible
Mefloquine	Pfmdr1 and others	Amplification in copy number of *pfmdr1*
Halofantrine	Pfmdr1 and others	Amplification in copy number of *pfmdr1*
Quinine	Pfmdr1 and others	Unclear but occasionally amplification in copy number of *pfmdr1* is seen

For key to the abbreviations see the text.

DRUGS ACTING TO PREVENT SYNTHESIS OF PYRIMIDINES

The synthesis of DNA, essential for parasite replication, requires both pyrimidine and purine nucleotides. Malarial parasites scavenge the purine bases from the host red blood cell but synthesize the pyrimidine bases de novo. Pyrimidine synthesis requires folate as a co-factor, as does the process of synthesis of the amino acids serine and methionine. Four groups of drugs (sulphonamides (usually sulphadoxine), sulphones (usually dapsone), pyrimethamine and proguanil) act at various points in the parasite pathway for folate production, the first part of this metabolic pathway being absent in man. Sulphonamides and sulphones inhibit the enzyme dihydropteroate synthetase (DHPS) that catalyses the linkage of *p*-aminobenzoic acid (PABA) to synthesize 7,8-dihydropteroate. Pyrimethamine and proguanil act further along the folate synthetic pathway by interfering with the reduction of dihydrofolate to tetrahydrofolate by dihydrofolate reductase (DHFR). These two groups of drugs are often used in combination to maximize the inhibitory effect.

The exact mechanism underlying *P. falciparum* resistance to sulphadoxine has not yet been definitively demonstrated and more than one mechanism may be involved including decreased drug uptake, the utilization of alternative pathways of synthesis and alteration of the target enzyme DHPS. Cloning studies of the DHPS gene have shown it to be a bifunctional gene, that in addition to encoding DHPS, it also encodes 6-hydroxylmethyl-7,8-dihydropterin pyrophosphokinase (PPPK), an enzyme that catalyses the previous step to DHPS in the folic acid synthetic pathway (Triglia and Cowman, 1994). Sequence analysis of the DHPS gene from sulphadoxine-sensitive and resistant parasites has shown amino acid differences that appear to be linked to the mechanism of resistance. This is similar to the findings in sulpha-resistant bacteria which express mutant forms of DHPS. However, until the mutant enzymes are synthesized and shown to be less easily inhibited by drug, the amino acid mutations must remain only the presumptive cause of drug resistance.

DHFR activity is inhibited by both the direct binding of pyrimethamine, which has a much higher affinity for the parasite form of the enzyme than the human form, and by the competitive binding of the folic acid antagonist cycloguanil, which is formed by the metabolism of proguanil in vivo. Resistance of the malaria parasite to both pyrimethamine and cycloguanil is widespread and develops rapidly once the drug is used in the field, suggesting that a single gene may be involved in conferring resistance. The gene for DHFR has been cloned and, as for DHPS, encodes a bifunctional enzyme complex: DHFR and thymidylate synthetase. Sequence analysis of a number of field isolates of *P. falciparum* that differ in their sensitivity to pyrimethamine and cycloguanil has revealed that particular mutations in the DHFR gene are linked to drug resistance. In contrast to the situation for DHPS, further studies have been performed that demonstrate that drug-resistant mutants do indeed have a lower affinity of binding for pyrimethamine. The most important amino acid change for pyrimethamine resistance has been shown to be that of serine to asparagine at position 108 in the parasite DHFR protein, which confers a ten-fold increase in resistance (Cowman et al, 1988). Subsequent changes at positions 52 or 58, such as the presence of cysteine at position 52, result in further increases in resistance to about 100-fold compared to sensitive isolates. Comparative crystal structures for DHFR of other organisms suggests that these amino acid changes are located in the active site of the enzyme.

Laboratory studies using high levels of drug to select resistant forms of rodent malarias and *P. falciparum* grown in vitro, suggest that resistance can also arise secondary to amplification of the DHFR gene and over-expression of the enzyme. However, there is no data to suggest that such a mechanism operates in the field.

Resistance to cycloguanil is also caused by a mutation that affects residue 108 of the DHFR protein, but in this case serine is changed to threonine (Foote et al, 1990a). A second mutation at position 16 is also present. Parasites that are resistant to both pyrimethamine and cycloguanil have been identified, and it appears that an extended set of three or four mutations is required, including a mutation at position 164 (Peterson et al, 1988). This requirement for additional mutations suggests that the combination of these two drugs may be useful in delaying the appearance of resistant forms.

RESISTANCE TO QUINOLINE-TYPE ANTI-MALARIALS

This group of drugs, which includes quinine, chloroquine, amodiaquine, mefloquine and halofantrine, have been the mainstay of anti-malarial chemotherapy. Resistance to chloroquine, the most widely used of these drugs, appears to have arisen in Asia and South America at about the same time in the early 1960s and then spread to all other continents. The mode of action of chloroquine appears to involve concentration of the drug in the food vacuole of the parasite, the major digestive organelle, in which red blood cell haemoglobin is metabolized. Metabolism of haemoglobin yields amino acids that are used for parasite protein synthesis but also free haem which is toxic to the parasite. This toxicity is prevented by polymerization of the haem into an insoluble pigment called haemozoin, which is harmless to the parasite. It seems likely, on current evidence, that chloroquine acts to prevent haem polymerization and hence accumulation of toxic haem compounds occurs in the food vacuole (Cowman and Karcz, 1993). The mechanism of resistance of malarial parasites to drugs such as chloroquine is also still controversial, but appears to be multigenic, a finding that would harmonize with the relatively long time required for resistance to develop in the field and the relatively few locations at which it has appeared independently.

Chloroquine-resistant malaria parasites accumulate less chloroquine than chloroquine-sensitive parasites, an observation that could be due to diminished uptake of drug by the parasite or increased efflux, or a combination of both effects. Although previous studies favoured the increased efflux hypothesis, and indeed sparked the search for molecules capable of pumping chloroquine out of cells, more recent data favours the model of decreased drug uptake by resistant parasites (Ginsburg and Stein, 1991). The most likely mechanism for impaired drug uptake is impaired acidification of the food vacuole, although the mechanism by which this occurs is by no means clear.

The chloroquine resistance phenotype in *P. falciparum* can be reversed by several compounds including verapamil, and a combination of chloroquine and desipramine can cure Aotus monkeys (*Aotus trivirgatus*) of a chloroquine-resistant *P. falciparum* infection. Resistance to quinine and other quinoline-type anti-malarials can also be decreased with verapamil and some other compounds. Unfortunately, for many of the compounds, the concentration of drug needed to achieve reversal of resistance causes toxic side effects. Research continues into reversal drugs or combinations that may be safely used in humans. The demonstration that the chloroquine resistance phenotype could be modulated by verapamil and the early reports of apparent rapid efflux were strongly reminiscent of the phenomenon of multi-drug resistance (MDR) of mammalian tumour cells to cytotoxic drugs. MDR in tumour cells is due to an ATP-dependent transport protein termed P-glycoprotein that is able to remove many chemically distinct anti-tumour drugs from the cell. Accordingly, researchers set out to determine whether *P. falciparum* possessed an analogue of P-glycoprotein, and two P-glycoprotein-like genes (*pfmdr1* and *pfmdr2*) were indeed found (Foote et al, 1989; Wilson et al, 1989).

The pfmdr1 protein, of 162 kDa, has a structure typical of the ATP-binding cassette (ABC) family of transporters that includes the P-glycoproteins and the cystic fibrosis transport regulator. Pfmdr1 has six putative transmembrane regions and one nucleotide binding fold, repeated in tandem. It is located on the membrane of the food vacuole, the organelle in which chloroquine accumulates. The pfmdr2 protein, in contrast, has ten putative transmembrane regions and only one nucleotide binding fold, a structure similar to a protein involved in heavy metal tolerance in yeast.

The multiple-drug resistance phenotype in tumour cells is associated with amplification of *mdr* genes and overexpression of the *mdr* gene product, also called P-glycoprotein (Gros et al, 1986). Although amplification of the *pfmdr1* gene has been found in some chloroquine-resistant *P. falciparum* field isolates, this is clearly not found in the majority of resistant isolates. Instead, there is a strong correlation between the presence of particular mutations and chloroquine resistance (Foote et al, 1990b). However, this correlation is not perfect, and several clearly resistant field isolates have the same *pfmdr1* gene sequence as found in sensitive isolates. The *pfmdr1* gene has been transfected into chinese hamster ovary (CHO) cells and causes a chloroquine-sensitive phenotype with increased accumulation of the drug into the acidic lysosomal compartment (van Es et al, 1994). If the CHO cells were transfected with the mutant form of *pfmdr1* found in some chloroquine-resistant isolates, the CHO cells were not sensitive to chloroquine and it was shown that the pH of the lysosomes was the same as in untransfected CHO cells. These experiments suggested that chloroquine resistance is related to accumulation of drug in the acidic vacuolar compartment and that mutations in the *pfmdr1* gene can influence the level of accumulation of the drug and hence the chloroquine resistance phenotype.

This seemingly clear state of affairs is greatly complicated by the experiments of Wellems et al (1991) who used genetic cross experiments to demonstrate that chloroquine resistance is associated with a single gene located in a specific region of chromosome 7. *pfmdr1* is found on chromosome 5 and was therefore not implicated in chloroquine resistance in these studies. Sequencing studies have not yet identified the candidate drug resistance gene on chromosome 7, but apparently have stumbled across one of the genes that encode the protein responsible for cytoadherence. It is reasonable to suggest that given the accumulated evidence concerning *pfmdr1* and its relation to chloroquine sensitivity, chloroquine resistance is due to the action of several gene products including that of *pfmdr1*, a locus on chromosome 7 and possibly a locus on chromosome 3 (Foote and Cowman, 1994). There is presently no convincing evidence to link *pfmdr2* expression to resistance to any anti-malarial drugs.

Experiments in which parasites were grown in in vitro culture in the presence of increasing concentrations of chloroquine had shown a decrease in mefloquine resistance at the same time as there was a decrease in the number of copies of *pfmdr1*. Conversely, selection for mefloquine resistance selects for an increase in the number of copies of the *pfmdr1* gene and also a decrease in the level of chloroquine resistance. Mefloquine-resistant parasites also appear to be more resistant to halofantrine and often quinine, and this relationship is also found in field isolates (Wilson et al, 1993).

Exactly how the *pfmdr1* gene is involved in mefloquine, halofantrine and quinine resistance has yet to be determined.

DIAGNOSIS OF MALARIA USING GENETIC TECHNIQUES

The microscopic diagnosis of malaria infection requires considerable skill, particularly if parasitaemia is low, as it can be in symptomatic non-immunes experiencing their first *P. falciparum* infection. Pathology services operating in non-endemic countries may only rarely encounter blood smears from patients where malaria is part of the differential diagnosis and may experience considerable difficulty in the correct interpretation of a thick blood film. Diagnosis by microscopy is also extremely time consuming, and for this reason many surveillance programmes in endemic countries have accumulated veritable mountains of unread malaria slides. The development of a sensitive, automatable diagnostic procedure that does not require specialized training of the operator has been a major objective of recent research efforts. Several tests including the quantitative blood count (QBC™), the HRP-II immunoassay (*Para*Sight^R-F™, see Chapter 4: The clinical manifestations and diagnosis of malaria, for further discussion of these tests) and various DNA and RNA-based assays have been evaluated in recent years. Ideally, such tests should be simple to perform, sensitive, rapid and, importantly for control programmes in developing countries, inexpensive.

In patients who lack any form of anti-malarial immunity, the detection of parasites in a febrile patient provides the definitive diagnosis of malaria. In contrast, individuals of all ages living in endemic areas, commonly have parasitaemias, and the mere detection of parasites, particularly in adults, does not necessarily provide a diagnosis for a febrile illness. Nevertheless, the presence of parasitaemia means that there is parasite genetic material present and tests have been developed to detect both parasite DNA and RNA in human blood. The presence of parasite genetic material is detected by the process of nucleic acid hybridization in which a particular probe sequence is reacted with the parasite material. Complementary sequences will hybridize by base pairing and the presence of the duplex structure detected by virtue of some sort of label attached to the probe sequence. The label may be radioactive such as ^{32}P or ^{35}S, or non-radioactive using more recently developed colorimetric or luminescent probes.

Sensitivity of DNA diagnostic tests may be increased in several ways. Firstly, if the target sequence occurs many times within the genome, such as in the case of repetitive elements, then each parasite will contribute a correspondingly greater number of target sequences. For this reason, almost all the early tests for *P. falciparum* malaria attempted to detect the presence of a 21 bp repetitive element present in subtelomeric repeats on all parasite chromosomes (Corcoran et al, 1988). This repeat is specific for *P. falciparum* and allows the detection of about 1000 parasites/sample. DNA based tests are capable of distinguishing between different species of *Plasmodium* using specially designed probes. In the case of repetitive element probes, DNA probes have only been described for *P. falciparum* and *P. vivax* and the vivax probe is less useful in detecting low parasitaemias (Barker, 1990). Alternative targets such as the genes encoding the small subunit ribosomal RNA may be used to design species-specific probes, and a method to detect all four malarial species that commonly infect man has been described (Snounou et al, 1993b).

The development of the polymerase chain reaction (PCR) gave a method for increasing the number of copies of any target sequence and could be used to increase the number of copies of the repetitive element, allowing a theoretical sensitivity of 1 parasite/sample. Practically this is rarely achieved, one of the reasons being that blood contains poorly defined substances that inhibit the PCR reaction and decrease the yield of product. Detection of levels of parasitaemia of 0.00002% and less have been reported in laboratory studies, but there have not been many examples of extensive trials either in the field or in hospital diagnostic departments. In one of the larger field trials, 229 samples from 48 patients living in an endemic area in Venezuela were examined for parasitaemia by a PCR reaction followed by hybridization with oligonucleotide probes. The sensitivity of PCR based diagnosis, compared to microscopy, was 78% and the specificity was 97% (Laserson et al, 1994). A second disadvantage of the PCR approach had been that high sensitivity required large numbers of cycles of amplification which could take many hours. Analysis required the running of an agarose gel which increased the time to diagnosis. The availability of thin tube PCR machines has dramatically shortened the time of the PCR reaction and alternative detection procedures may make this approach feasible for diagnosis of acute infections. Finally, the results of PCR tests are prone to inaccuracies resulting from contamination between samples and scrupulous precautions need to be in place to avoid this.

An alternative diagnostic approach of some interest is to use probes that detect the ribosomal RNA of parasites (Waters and McCutchan, 1989). Ribosomal RNA is an extremely abundant cellular component being present in 10–50 times greater amounts than DNA with all of the RNA being available as target compared to the small percentage of DNA that exists as a specific target sequence. Species specific probes have been developed and the test shows promise under laboratory conditions detecting parasitaemias in the order of 0.0005% (Lal et al, 1989; Waters and McCutchan, 1989). As yet there is little data on the stability of RNA in field samples or its sensitivity in large numbers of patients.

The availability of sensitive tests for detection of parasite DNA may also be used in various epidemiological contexts. The analysis of mosquitoes for the species of malaria that they carry is now feasible as is a form of contact tracing in which polymorphic antigen sequences are used to follow man–mosquito contact throughout a community (Snounou et al, 1993a). The availability of highly sensitive tests for detection of parasitaemia will demonstrate a higher prevalence both of infection and mixed infection by different parasite strains and species. The significance of this for our understanding of immunity and the criteria for demonstrable vaccine efficacy is major.

FUTURE DIRECTIONS

Future molecular biological experimentation will focus on several areas of inquiry. The genetic mapping project will continue in its aim of providing a complete physical map of the *P. falciparum* genome, as well as a complete linkage map of yeast artificial chromosome clones. The next milestone will be the mapping of transcriptional units for the different life cycle stages as well as the placement on the map of all known genes and sequence tagged sites. The complete sequencing of the genome should eventually follow but will require substantial funds and it is not at all clear that any major funding agency currently views such an undertaking with sufficient enthusiasm.

Biological problems of outstanding interest such as the mechanism of invasion of the red blood cell, the genetic basis of antigenic variation and the structure of the cytoadherence ligand will be the focus of much work. Many merozoite proteins have been identified but their functions and the interactions between them remain enigmatic. Similarly, the cloning of *Plasmodium falciparum* erythrocyte membrane protein-1 (Pf-EMP-1) if not already a reality, is expected to provide insights into the mechanism by which infected red blood cells adhere to vascular endothelial cell receptors and initiate the process of cerebral malaria.

Efforts at the production of a malaria vaccine will continue and the identification and expression of putative host protective molecules from all life cycle stages will continue apace. Formidable problems in producing proteins, protein fragments and peptides of the correct conformation and immunogenicity exist, as do the correct combination of components to provide immunity against all stages of the parasite. The development of DNA vaccines suggests a powerful means of shortening this process. The recognition that much of the toxic effect of parasites is due to action of host cytokines released in response to parasite molecules such as glycolipids has opened new approaches to the development of anti-disease vaccines. Identification of parasite molecules that stimulate the release of cytokines, and the elucidation of mechanisms that are responsible for down-regulation of cytokine release in immune individuals, may facilitate novel prophylactic and therapeutic interventions that prevent the more severe forms of disease of *P. falciparum* and other species.

Research into drug resistance mechanisms will continue, but more effort needs to be devoted to the identification of parasite-specific metabolic pathways that may be amenable to inhibition by existing or novel agents. A particularly exciting possibility may be the development of inhibitors of the action of transcription factors so that antigenic variation is prevented. This would significantly decrease the pathogenicity of parasite strains.

It is likely that refinements to diagnostic procedures based on PCR will occur. However, their utility for diagnostic use will depend on how widely used PCR diagnostic procedures become in general pathological practice. The success of antibody-based detection methods, such as the HRP-II dipstick, together with the advantage of a portable procedure not requiring instrumentation, reduces the need for PCR-based tests. Of considerable value would be the development of a test that is able to determine whether, in an endemic area, a pyrexial individual with parasitaemia is suffering from malaria. Perhaps such a test will need to determine simultaneously the presence of malaria parasites and cytokine releasing molecules of parasite origin, as well as the level of host cytokines such as tumour necrosis factor (TNF) and the level of host antibodies that block parasite-induced cytokine release.

The holy grail of recent research has been the development of a transformation system for the parasite that would allow the inactivation of parasite genes and the introduction of exogenous genes (Goonewardene et al, 1993). This approach is extremely powerful in defining gene function and could be used to dissect the involvement of parasite proteins in complex phenomena such as invasion process and chloroquine resistance. Finally, research will continue into the development of transgenic mosquitoes that are poor vectors for the transmission of malaria. Such a development has the capacity of aiding malaria control over geographical expanses but must first be subject to extremely strict regulatory safeguards and environmental testing before any consideration of widespread release may be entertained. The take home message is that no 'magic bullets' are yet available as a result of the efforts of the genetic engineers and conventional approaches of drug prophylaxis and therapy, vector control and man–mosquito contact avoidance will have to suffice for the present.

SUMMARY

The search for a vaccine against malaria has led to a concerted effort to understand the structure and function of many malaria proteins, as well as their capacity to induce host protective responses. The numerous constraints of working with the various malarial species has spurred the early and widespread adoption of the techniques of recombinant DNA technology. Consequently, we know a great deal about the primary structure of many malarial proteins, particularly those of *P. falciparum*. In particular, we know a great deal about the variant forms of several important vaccine candidates such as the merozoite proteins MSP-1, MSP-2 and AMA-1, information that will be useful for the formulation of vaccines that can be used worldwide. Less is known about the function of these proteins, and this remains an urgent need if new therapies aimed at interfering with key parasitic processes such as invasion of red cells and cytoadherence are to be developed. A great deal of effort has been expended in developing expression and delivery systems that can produce malarial proteins in abundant amounts and in the correct conformation, in order to induce effective, high titre immune responses reliably in people with diverse histocompatability status. The recent development of DNA-based vaccines appears particularly promising. Significant advances have been made in our understanding of the mechanisms of parasite resistance to drugs, although development of new drug targets has been less successful. A recently inaugurated malaria genome project is taking the first steps towards providing a complete physical map of the malaria genome and ultimately the complete genomic sequence. Notwithstanding the many insights provided by molecular biological studies of parasites, the conventional armoury of drugs and control programmes of various sorts appears likely to remain our major defence against malaria for some time to come.

Acknowledgements

This work is supported by funds from the National Health and Medical Research Council and the National Institutes of Health grant DK32094–10.

REFERENCES

Anderson RM & May RM (1991) *Infectious Diseases of Humans: Dynamics and Control.* Oxford: Oxford University Press.

Barker RH (1990) DNA probe diagnosis of parasitic infections. *Experimental Parasitology* **70:** 494–499.

Coppel RL, Davern KM & McConville MJ (1994) Immunochemistry of parasite antigens. In van Oss CJ & van Regenmortel MHV (eds) *Immunochemistry*, pp 475–532. New York: Marcel Dekker Inc.

Corcoran LM, Thompson JK, Walliker D & Kemp DJ (1988) Homologous recombination within subtelomeric repeat sequences generates chromosome size polymorphisms in *Plasmodium falciparum. Cell* **53:** 807–813.

Cowman AF & Foote SJ (1990) Chemotherapy and drug resistance in malaria. *International Journal of Parasitology* **20:** 503–513.

Cowman AF & Karcz S (1993) Drug resistance and the P-glycoprotein homologues of *Plasmodium falciparum. Seminars in Cell Biology* **4:** 29–35.

Cowman AF, Morry MJ, Biggs BA et al (1988) Amino acid changes linked to pyrimethamine resistance in the dihydrofolate reductase-thymidylate synthase gene of *Plasmodium falciparum. Proceedings of the National Academy of Sciences of the USA* **85:** 9109–9113.

Foote SJ & Kemp DJ (1989) Chromosomes of malarial parasites. *Trends in Genetics* **5:** 337–342.

Foote SJ & Cowman AF (1994) The mode of action and the mechanism of resistance to antimalarial drugs. *Acta Tropica* **56:** 157–171.

Foote SJ, Thompson JK, Cowman AF & Kemp DJ (1989) Amplification of the multidrug resistance gene in some chloroquine-resistant isolates of *Plasmodium falciparum. Cell* **57:** 921–930.

Foote SJ, Galatis D & Cowman AF (1990a) Amino acids in the dihydrofolate reductase-thymidylate synthase gene of *Plasmodium falciparum* involved in cycloguanil resistance differ from those involved in pyrimethamine resistance. *Proceedings of the National Academy of Sciences of the USA* **87:** 3014–3017.

Foote SJ, Kyle DE, Martin RK, et al (1990b) Several alleles of the multidrug-resistance gene are closely linked to chloroquine resistance in *Plasmodium falciparum. Nature* **345:** 255–258.

Gardner MJ, Feagin JE, Moore DJ et al (1993) Sequence and organization of large subunit rRNA genes from the extrachromosomal 35 kb circular DNA of the malaria parasite *Plasmodium falciparum. Nucleic Acids Research* **21:** 1067–1071.

Ginsburg H & Stein WD (1991) Kinetic modelling of chloroquine uptake by malaria-infected erythrocytes. Assessment of the factors that may determine drug resistance. *Biochemical Pharmacology* **41:** 1463–1470.

Goonewardene R, Daily J, Kaslow D, et al (1993) Transfection of the malaria parasite and expression of firefly luciferase. *Proceedings of the National Academy of Sciences of the USA* **90:** 5234–5236.

Gros P, Croop J & Housman D (1986) Mammalian multidrug resistance gene: complete cDNA sequence indicates strong homology to bacterial transport proteins. *Cell* **47:** 371–380.

Howard RJ & Pasloske BL (1993) Target antigens for asexual malaria vaccine development. *Parasitology Today* **9:** 369–372.

Kemp DJ, Coppel RL & Anders RF (1987) Repetitive proteins and genes of malaria. *Annual Reviews in Microbiology* **41**: 181–208.

Lal AA, Changkasiri S, Hollingdale MR & McCutchan TF (1989) Ribosomal RNA-based diagnosis of *Plasmodium falciparum* malaria. *Molecular and Biochemical Parasitology* **36**: 67–72.

Lanzer M, Debruin D, Wertheimer SP & Ravetch JV (1994) Organization of chromosomes in *Plasmodium falciparum* – a model for generating karyotypic diversity. *Parasitology Today* **10**: 114–117.

Laserson KF, Petralanda I, Hamlin DM, et al (1994) Use of the polymerase chain reaction to directly detect malaria parasites in blood samples from the Venezuelan amazon. *American Journal of Tropical Medicine and Hygiene* **50**: 169–180.

Murphy G, Basri H, Purnomo et al (1993) Vivax malaria resistant to treatment and prophylaxis with chloroquine. *Lancet* **341**: 96–100.

Pancake SJ, Holt GD, Mellouk S & Hoffman SL (1992) Malaria sporozoites and circumsporozoite proteins bind specifically to sulphated glycoconjugates. *Journal of Cellular Biochemistry* **117**: 1351–1357.

Peterson DS, Walliker D & Wellems TE (1988) Evidence that a point mutation in dihydrofolate reductase-thymidylate synthase confers resistance to pyrimethamine in falciparum malaria. *Proceedings of the National Academy of Sciences of the USA* **85**: 9114–9118.

Roberts DJ, Biggs BA, Brown G & Newbold CI (1993) Protection, pathogenesis and phenotypic plasticity in *Plasmodium falciparum* malaria. *Parasitology Today* **9**: 281–286.

Scherf A & Mattei D (1992) Cloning and characterization of chromosome breakpoints of *Plasmodium falciparum*: breakage and new telomere formation occurs frequently and randomly in sub-telomeric genes. *Nucleic Acids Research* **20**: 1491–1496.

Schwartz DC & Cantor CR (1984) Separation of yeast chromosome-sized DNAs by pulsed field gradient gel electrophoresis. *Cell* **37**: 67–75.

Sedegah M, Hedstrom R, Hobart P & Hoffman SL (1994) Protection against malaria by immunization with plasmid DNA encoding circumsporozoite protein. *Proceedings of the National Academy of Sciences of the USA* **91**: 9866–9870.

Snounou G, Pinheiro L, Goncalves A et al (1993a) The importance of sensitive detection of malaria parasites in the human and insect hosts in epidemiological studies, as shown by the analysis of field samples from Guinea Bissau. *Transactions of the Royal Society of Tropical Medicine and Hygeine* **87**: 649–653.

Snounou G, Viriyakosol S, Jarra W et al (1993b) Identification of the four human malaria parasite species in field samples by the polymerase chain reaction and detection of a high prevalence of mixed infections. *Molecular and Biochemical Parasitology* **58**: 283–292.

Triglia T & Cowman AF (1994) Primary structure and expression of the dihydropteroate synthetase gene of *Plasmodium falciparum*. *Proceedings of the National Academy of Sciences of the USA* **91**: 7149–7153.

Triglia T, Wellems TE & Kemp DJ (1992) Towards a high resolution map of the *Plasmodium falciparum* genome. *Parasitology Today* **8**: 225–229.

van Es HHG, Karcz S, Chu F, et al (1994) Expression of the plasmodial pfmdr1 gene in mammalian cells is associated with increased susceptibility to chloroquine. *Molecular and Cellular Biology* **14**: 2419–2428.

Waters AP (1994) The ribosomal RNA genes of *Plasmodium*. *Advances in Parasitology* **34**: 246–250.

Waters AP & McCutchan TF (1989) Rapid, sensitive diagnosis of malaria based on ribosomal RNA. *Lancet* **i**: 1343–1346.

Weber JL (1988) Molecular biology of malaria parasites. *Experimental Parasitology* **66**: 143–170.

Weber JL (1989) Molecular biology of malaria parasites. *Experimental Parasitology* **68**: 373 (Erratum).

Wellems TE, Walker JA & Panton LJ (1991) Genetic mapping of the chloroquine-resistance locus on *Plasmodium falciparum* chromosome 7. *Proceedings of the National Academy of Sciences of the USA* **88**: 3382–3386.

Wilson CM, Serrano AE, Wasley A et al (1989) Amplification of a gene related to mammalian mdr genes in drug-resistant *Plasmodium falciparum*. *Science* **244**: 1184–1186.

Wilson CM, Volkman SK, Thaithong S et al (1993) Amplification of *pfmdr1* associated with mefloquine and halofantrine resistance in *Plasmodium falciparum* from Thailand. *Molecular and Biochemical Parasitology* **57**: 151–160.

9

The biology of malarial fever

DOMINIC KWIATKOWSKI

A critical discovery in the biology of malaria was the observation that the clinical symptoms are directly linked to the replicative cycle of the parasite within host erythrocytes (Golgi, 1889). Patients with malaria experience paroxysms of fever that recur periodically as successive cohorts of erythrocytic schizonts rupture, in their billions, to release their progeny. The mechanism of the fever was obscure until relatively recently and is still lacking in many of the molecular details. However, it is now fairly certain that malaria fever is mediated by pyrogenic cytokines such as tumour necrosis factor (TNF), produced by the host in response to schizont rupture, which act on the hypothalamus to promote the physiological elevation of body temperature. The recognition that fever has a molecular mechanism has served to highlight the fact that it is a natural host response to infection, and that it may serve some biological purpose.

FEVER AS A PHYSIOLOGICAL RESPONSE TO INFECTION

Humans are able to maintain a stable body temperature despite huge fluctuations in their level of activity and in climate. This homeostatic *tour de force* entails continual physiological and behavioural adjustments that are coordinated by a thermoregulatory centre in the anterior hypothalamus (for a review, see Kluger, 1979). It is only in extreme conditions that the hypothalamic control of body temperature breaks down and the individual becomes hyperthermic. This is not the case with fever, where the hypothalamus retains control. Fever is an adjustment of the body's thermostat to a higher set-point, and the thermoregulatory centre works to maintain temperature at precisely this point. This is illustrated by the sensations that people experience during an acute episode of fever. At the onset there is a transient discrepancy between actual temperature and the new thermoregulatory set-point, so the individual suddenly feels cold and shivery. As a result of shivering and other physiological changes, as well as behavioural responses such as wrapping up warm, body temperature soon rises to the higher set-point and the individual no longer feels cold. During the next phase, if the febrile stimulus remains constant, the affected individual may be unaware that their body temperature is high. When the stimulus of the fever declines, the set-point returns to normal. Now the

371

sensation is reversed, because actual temperature is suddenly higher than the set-point so the individual feels hot and perspires profusely. Malaria fever paroxysms clearly illustrate this sequence of events. They begin with chills and intense shivering, known as rigors, which cease once the temperature has reached a high level, and the paroxysm terminates with a phase of profuse perspiration known as defervescence.

The mechanism of infectious fever has become much clearer in the past decade, mainly due to molecular biological advances that have identified the key mediators. Fever occurs when the microbe triggers the host to release specific polypeptides that act on the brain to cause fever. These molecules are classically called 'endogenous pyrogens'. Monocytes and macrophages appear to be the dominant source, but they can also be produced by other cell types. They are a subset of the family of small polypeptides known as cytokines, which act as messengers between different parts of the immune system. Endogenous pyrogen is a term reserved for those cytokines that act directly on the anterior hypothalamus to alter the thermoregulatory set-point, probably by virtue of their ability to induce prostaglandin E_2 synthesis in that environment. There is still some debate about exactly which cytokines possess this property (Dinarello, 1987; Kluger, 1991) but tumour necrosis factor (TNF), interleukin-1β (IL-1β), interleukin-1α (IL-1α), interleukin-6 (IL-6) and interferon-α are generally supposed to be authentic endogenous pyrogens, while other candidates include lymphotoxin-α (LT-α) and macrophage inflammatory protein-1 (MIP-1).

Elevated temperature is only part of the clinical syndrome of fever, which is typically associated with body aches, anorexia and sleepiness, plus weight loss if the fever is chronic. TNF and IL-1 possess physiological and metabolic properties that can account for most of these symptoms (Beutler and Cerami, 1989; Dinarello, 1991). They also elicit acute phase responses such as neutrophilia and hypoferraemia, while IL-6 stimulates the synthesis of acute phase proteins. At a more local level, TNF and IL-1 act to recruit inflammatory cells to sites of infection or injury by stimulating vascular endothelium to express adhesion molecules which attract circulating leukocytes and platelets. Most importantly, they activate various compartments of the immune system: IL-1 in particular acts as a positive cofactor in the response of B- and T-cells to antigen stimulation, while both TNF and IL-1 promote phagocytosis and the production of reactive intermediates by neutrophils and macrophages. Thus fever should be viewed as part of a package of inflammatory and immunologic changes rather than as an isolated elevation of body temperature.

It is remarkable how little is known about why animals raise their body temperature in response to infection. This response has been conserved throughout vertebrate evolution despite its huge cost in terms of metabolic energy, implying that it serves some biological purpose (Kluger, 1979). The best evidence for this comes from classical studies in desert iguanas. When infected with certain bacteria, these animals normally raise their temperature by migrating to a warmer environment, and if they are prevented from doing so then the infection has a higher mortality rate. In mammals the evidence is more circumstantial, and rests largely on the observation that febrile temperatures augment immunological functions such as lymphocyte proliferation and neutrophil chemotaxis (Roberts, 1991). Febrile temperatures can also directly inhibit the proliferation of certain microbes in vitro, and *Plasmodium falciparum* provides a clear example of this effect (Kwiatkowski, 1989). This latter observation, coupled with the evolutionary argument, raises the possibility that fever benefits the malaria-infected individual.

CYTOKINES INVOLVED IN MALARIA FEVER

Before focusing on malaria it is worth noting that although the causal relationship between cytokine production and fever has been clearly demonstrated in a variety of experimental models, it is technically much more difficult to prove that naturally occuring fever is due to the action of a specific cytokine or group of cytokines (Kluger, 1991). Preliminary evidence that endogenous pyrogens are involved in malaria fever was obtained well before these mediators had been defined at the molecular level, by collecting patients' blood while their temperature was rising rapidly and re-injecting it after the malaria had been treated (Cranston, 1966). This type of investigation became much easier with the advent of sensitive cytokine assays, and over the past few years there have been numerous reports of high circulating cytokine levels in patients with malaria fever. The challenge has been to prove that this cytokine response is the cause of the fever. This has largely been achieved, in that there is now reasonably robust evidence that TNF is a critical mediator of malaria fever, while there is circumstantial evidence that other cytokines also play a role.

There have been at least nine independent reports of high TNF levels in plasma or serum of malaria-infected individuals (Scuderi et al, 1986 ; Kern et al, 1989; Grau et al, 1989; Kwiatkowski et al, 1989, 1990; Butcher et al, 1990; Molyneux et al, 1991; Shaffer et al, 1991; Karunaweera et al, 1992b) TNF is unquestionably a potent pyrogen (Dinarello et al, 1986), and three lines of evidence indicate that it has a causal role in the pathogenesis of malaria fever. First, it is well established that the fever is associated with schizont rupture (Golgi, 1889), and in vitro studies show that this event triggers a burst of TNF release from human monocytes (Kwiatkowski et al, 1989). Second, malaria fever is accompanied, or slightly preceded, by a sharp elevation of circulating TNF levels. This relationship has been difficult to investigate in falciparum malaria because of its irregular fever pattern, but it has been elegantly demonstrated during the discrete fever paroxysms of *P. vivax* infection (Karunaweera et al, 1992b). Finally, therapeutic studies with monoclonal anti-TNF antibodies in cerebral malaria have produced clear evidence that fever is reduced when TNF bioactivity is inhibited (Kwiatkowski et al, 1993).

Other endogenous pyrogens are also released into circulation during clinical attacks of malaria, including IL-Iβ (Cannon et al, 1988), IL-6 (Kern, et al, 1989; Molyneux et al, 1991), IL-1α (Kwiatkowski et al, 1990) and LT-α (Clark et al, 1992). In addition, there are elevated levels of interferon-γ (IFN-γ) (Kwiatkowski et al, 1990) and IL-2, which probably contribute to fever by promoting the production of authentic endogenous pyrogens (Dinarello, 1987). None of these cytokines have so far been subject to the same level of scrutiny as TNF, and it is difficult to appraise their contribution to malaria fever by simply comparing their plasma levels, as they vary in their circulating half-life and their ease of measurement (Dinarello and Cannon, 1993). Moreover, the abundance of a cytokine may be of less significance than its position in the cytokine cascade. For example, IL-6 is of interest because it is a potent endogenous pyrogen and because it circulates at high levels in acute malaria, but it is also clear that TNF provides a major stimulus for IL-6 production (and not vice versa) so it is possible that the IL-6 response is largely dependent on a preceding TNF response. Because of the labyrinthine complexity of the cytokine network, researchers are increasingly turning to transgenic models in orders to define the role of specific cytokines in vivo. It is unfortunate that malaria fever is not amenable to this type of investigation, as fever is absent in experimental murine models of the infection.

In summary, it is presently uncertain to what extent malaria fever depends on cytokines other than TNF. This will become clearer once we have a better understanding of the precise mechanism by which schizont rupture induces cytokine production, and as more information becomes available about the clinical effects of specific cytokine inhibitors in severe malaria.

EVIDENCE FOR A MAJOR MALARIA TOXIN

Over 80 years ago Sir Ronald Ross wrote that '. . . it is now almost certain that (malaria) fever is connected with the discharge of some toxic substance from each mature sporoid at the moment when its spores are scattered in the serum' (Ross, 1911). This pyrogenic toxin receives frequent mention in the early malaria literature but the topic fell into neglect until it became apparent that much of malaria pathology could be explained by the ability of the parasite to induce specific cytokines. There is now considerable interest in the parasite component(s) that are responsible for stimulating the production of TNF and other endogenous pyrogens, not only because these are the putative stimuli of malaria fever but also because of the part they may play in severe malarial pathology, as discussed below. Definitions are important when speaking of toxins, because toxicity can arise through a multitude of mechanisms. The term 'malaria toxin' has classically been used to describe the putative fever-inducing component(s) of the parasite, and that is the sense in which it is used here.

Sporadic attempts to characterize the malaria toxin were made in the first half of the century. One of the earliest of these aimed to show that a major component of the toxin was malarial pigment. Crystalline hematin from uninfected erythrocytes was solubilized and injected into rabbits, who developed fever about an hour later (Brown, 1912). This finding was challenged by subsequent investigators (Morrison and Anderson, 1942) but even if correct, it is of doubtful relevance as it is now known that malarial pigment is a unique polymer of haem groups linked by an iron-carboxylate bond, known as hemozoin, which would have been absent from Brown's erythrocyte extracts (Slater et al, 1991). However, that is not the end of the story because recent studies show that particles of true malaria pigment, extracted from erythrocytes infected with *P. falciparum*, stimulate a strong TNF response when they are ingested by human monocytes (Pichyangkul et al, 1994). It is unclear how much of this TNF-inducing activity is due to hemozoin itself, and how much is due to proteins and lipids that tend to associate with the hemozoin. Pichyangkul and colleagues found that most of the TNF-inducing activity was removed from native pigment particles after protease digestion. On the other hand, it has been demonstrated that TNF is released when macrophages ingest highly purified native hemozoin or chemically synthesized hemozoin (B. Sherry and A. Cerami, personal communication). Taken together, these findings suggest that pigment particles induce TNF by virtue of their hemozoin composition and also due to some other active moiety, linked to polypeptide, that binds to the hemozoin.

   Another early idea was that the malaria toxin might resemble bacterial lipopolysaccharide (endotoxin). A number of investigations used the *Limulus* amoebocyte lysate (LAL) assay to detect circulating endotoxin-like substances in malaria patients. Some succeeded (Tubbs, 1980) but most did not (Glew and Levin, 1975; Greenwood et al, 1975). Parasite lysates were also found to be LAL-negative (Felton et al, 1980), and it was concluded that an endotoxin-like structure was unlikely to be responsible for malaria fever. The idea was revived when it was found that certain anti-gens extracted from *P. falciparum* culture supernatants were LAL-reactive (Jakobsen et al, 1988) and able to induce TNF and IL-6 production by monocytes and macrophages (Taverne, et al, 1990; Jakobsen et al, 1991; Johnson et al, 1993). This LAL-reactive component was found to be bound up in soluble antigen complex containing two merozoite proteins, but its composition has yet to be identified.

   There have also been reports of TNF induction by other malaria antigens (Picot et al, 1993). Such observations might suggest that the toxin is a complex mixture of substances rather than a specific entity. However, a growing body of data seems to contradict this view. Though there is no doubt that malaria parasites can induce TNF by various mechanisms, it appears that the bulk of the TNF-inducing activity of rupturing schizonts resides within a single molecule or a closely related family of molecules.

   The evidence for this stems from studies of TNF-induction by lysates of the rodent parasite *P. yoelii* (Bate et al, 1988, 1991). These investigators found that TNF release appeared to depend on a phospholipid structure, in that the activity of crude parasite lysates was greatly reduced after treatment with either phospholipase C, or mild alkali (a deacylating procedure), or hydrofluoric acid (which causes dephosphorylation). A phosphatidyl-inositol (PI)-like moiety was suggested by the observation that the activity was strongly inhibited in the presence of either PI derivatives (Bate et al, 1992c) or anti-PI antibodies (Bate et al, 1992a). Subsequent work showed that nanomolar concentrations of monoclonal antibodies (mAbs) which recognize PI can deplete the TNF-inducing activity of crude lysates of *P. falciparum* by over 95% (Bate and Kwiatkowski, 1994a). This investigation found that the same mAb can inhibit TNF-induction by disparate strains of *P. falciparum*, complementing the observation that antisera raised against lysates of *P. yoelii* can inhibit the TNF-inducing activity of *P. falciparum* and *P. vivax* (Bate et al, 1992b). Taken together, these results point to a major TNF-inducing toxin whose biological activity depends on a PI-like moiety which is relatively conserved among different plasmodial strains and species.

One interpretation of these observations is that the toxin may be a glycosylphosphatidylinositol (GPI) molecule. The major merozoite surface proteins (MSP-1 and MSP-2) and several other malarial proteins are co-valently linked to GPI anchors (Haldar et al, 1985; Braun-Breton et al, 1988; Smythe et al, 1988) and the biosynthesis of GPI precursors in *P. falciparum* has recently been described (Gerold et al, 1993). The primary function of GPI anchors is to provide a means of protein attachment to the plasma membrane, but in the higher eukaryotes there is also evidence that they can participate in signal transduction (Ferguson, 1994). Evidence for the GPI hypothesis came from a study where myristate- and palmitate-labelled forms of MSP-1 and MSP-2 from *P. falciparum* were affinity-purified, and shown to possess TNF-inducing activity which was lost when the acylated moiety was chemically or enzymatically cleaved (Schofield and Hackett, 1993). These results indicate that certain GPI molecules induce TNF, though they do not reveal what fraction of the total TNF-inducing activity of the parasite can be thus explained.

To conclude this section, there is evidence that a principal malaria toxin exists and a strong hint that it is related to GPI, but the biochemistry of the active component is not known with any certainty. It could even be a modified host structure, for it has been shown that TNF-inducing factors with broadly similar properties are present (albeit at much lower levels of activity) in lysates of uninfected erythrocytes (Bate and Kwiatkowski, 1994b). Given the efforts being made to purify the toxin and to submit it to formal structural analysis, hopefully these uncertainties will soon be resolved.

ANTI-PARASITIC EFFECTS OF THE FEVER RESPONSE

If malaria fever is considered as a physiological entity, where bouts of elevated temperature are the outward manifestation of a paroxysmal out-pouring of TNF and other cytokines, its potential role in host defence is immediately apparent. Evidence of the protective effects of TNF in malaria can be traced back to experiments where mice treated with bacterial endo-toxin were found to have increased resistance to *P. berghei* infection (Martin et al, 1967; MacGregor et al, 1969). Ian Clark was instrumental in developing the concept of a parasite toxin that induces macrophage-derived mediators with both anti-parasitic and pathological properties (Clark et al, 1981). The anti-malarial effects of crude preparations of TNF prompted

Playfair and colleagues to argue that a more appropriate name for this cytokine might be 'plasmodium necrosis factor', because, unlike tumours, malaria causes huge mortality before reproductive age and '. . . any rapidly produced substance that had a significant slowing effect on the acute growth rate of the blood-stage infection would therefore be intensely selected for' (Playfair et al, 1984). Once the gene had been cloned, it was shown that infusions of recombinant TNF could suppress parasite growth in murine malaria models (Clark et al, 1987b; Taverne et al, 1987) and that anti-TNF antibodies had the opposite effect (Neifer et al, 1989). Further evidence of the anti-malarial effects of TNF have come from studies of mice with constitutively elevated production owing to a human TNF transgene targeted to their T-lymphocytes (Taverne et al, 1994).

In vitro experiments reveal that TNF acts not by killing parasites directly, but by activating other effector mechanisms (Jensen et al, 1987; Taverne et al, 1987). Febrile temperatures are remarkably effective at suppressing the growth of *P. falciparum* in vitro, but as fever is difficult to study in mice it has received little attention as a potential effector mechanism. Macrophages and neutrophils exhibit various anti-malarial effects on stimulation with TNF and IL-1, including enhanced phagocytosis (Kumaratilake et al, 1991; Taverne et al , 1994) together with release of free oxygen radicals (Allison and Eugui, 1982; Clark and Hunt, 1983; Dockrell and Playfair, 1983, 1984; Ockenhouse and Shear, 1984; Wozencraft et al, 1984; Stocker et al, 1985; Clark et al, 1987a; Nnalue and Friedman, 1988) and nitric oxide (Rockett et al, 1991, 1992). Also, during fever paroxysms, the serum contains unidentified factors that synergize with TNF in killing sexual stage parasites (Karunaweera et al, 1992a).

While there is little doubt that paroxysms of malaria fever are associated with a burst of anti-parasitic activity, what is the evidence that this exerts a significant effect on the course of infection? And if fever does have an impact, how does this compare with other immune mechanisms that are believed to act on the asexual erythrocytic stage of parasite growth? These other mechanisms can be considered in two parts. A relatively early component depends on IFN-γ-secreting lymphocytes (the Th1 subset), which exert an important constraint on parasite growth, probably largely due to their ability to stimulate macrophages to kill parasites with nitric oxide, though this fails to cure the infection (Meding and Langhorne, 1991; Taylor-Robinson et al, 1993). A later component is the antibody response (dependent on the Th2 subset), which takes many weeks to mature but is essential for the eradication of parasites. This is a highly simplistic summary of how immunity to erythrocytic stage parasites is thought to be acquired in mice infected with *P. chabaudi chabaudi,* a model which parallels the human infection in several respects (though fever is absent). If we assume that similar mechanisms operate in man, then the initial question can be rephrased: what part does fever play in human malarial immunity, compared to an early Th1 response and a more slowly evolving antibody response?

Though there are very few quantitative immunological data which address this question, some strong clues are provided by observations of the natural history of malaria. Nowadays this would be difficult to study for ethical reasons, but it was described in considerable detail during the first half of the century because malaria was then used as a form of treatment for neurosyphilis. These classical data show that fever appears early in the course of infection and wanes long before parasites disappear from the blood. In other words, fever clearly plays no part in the eradication of infection. The most interesting aspect of fever is its relationship to parasite growth in the initial phase of infection. For the first few days after parasites emerge from the liver into the blood, the infected individual is asymptomatic, and during this time parasite density grows exponentially. Fever occurs as soon as parasite density exceeds a threshold level, typically around 100 parasites/μl in *P. vivax* infection or 10 000/μl for *P. falciparum* (Kitchen, 1949). Shortly after this, parasite density ceases to rise any further. In non-immune subjects it may then remain at a fairly constant level for several weeks, accompanied by periodic bouts of fever. It has been proposed that this early control of parasite growth can be largely attributed to the fever response (Kwiatkowski and Greenwood, 1989; Kwiatkowski, 1991; Kwiatkowski and Nowak, 1991). Here 'fever' is taken to mean not only elevated temperature (though this probably exerts a significant antiparasitic effect) but also the associated cytokine response.

This idea of fever as a regulator of parasite growth is quite compatible with the proposed role of the Th1 response, which presumably comes into play at about the same time (or shortly afterwards), as the macrophage-activating effects of TNF and IL-1 tend to be markedly augmented in the presence of IFN-γ. However, there are certain aspects of the fever response which can be clearly distinguished from a conventional T lymphocyte response, particularly in respect of its dynamical properties. The fever response requires no prior exposure or immunological memory; its antiparasitic actions are prompt and of short duration; and it is density-dependent (meaning that the strength of the response is largely determined by the current level of parasite density). These three attributes mean that the fever response is, at least in theory, capable of regulating the infection such that the parasite achieves a stable parasite population density: the principle is essentially the same as a domestic thermostat (Kwiatkowski, 1991). By contrast, conventional T- and B cell effector mechanisms lag at least a few days behind the antigenic stimulus, a situation much less likely to generate stable parasitaemia. These are of course blanket statements and there may be exceptions, e.g. in the $\gamma\delta$-T cell response. However, it is possible to draw the general conclusion that the dynamical properties of the fever response could explain the remarkable ability of human malaria parasites to achieve a stable population density through many cycles of parasite replication in a non-immune individual. Conversely, the less stable population dynamics observed in experimental models of murine malaria may be partly explained by the lack of a comparable density-dependent mechanism in these unnatural host–parasite combinations.

Though febrile temperatures are inhibitory to all stages of parasite development within the asexual erythrocytic cycle, the effect is strongest for older parasites (Kwiatkowski, 1989). An intriguing consequence is that fever probably acts to synchronize the parasite population, and this may in turn explain why malaria fever is often highly periodic. Mathematical considerations suggest that such effects are less likely to be observed for a parasite with a high replication rate, which may account for the fact that *P. falciparum* is the species least likely to generate a regular fever pattern (Kwiatkowski and Nowak, 1991).

DELETERIOUS EFFECTS OF EXCESSIVE CYTOKINE PRODUCTION

One of the dominant themes to have emerged from the cytokine literature of the past 10 years is that these molecules are involved both in host defence and in the pathology of infectious disease. This is not as paradoxical as it seems, for the value of the pro-inflammatory cytokines lies in their ability to initiate a cascade of inflammatory processes directed against a broad range of pathogens. Their lack of specificity is fundamental to their defensive role in the immunologically naive individual, but it carries the danger of damaging host tissues in the process of attacking the microbes.

As discussed earlier, generating cytokines that elicit fever is part of the normal host response to infection. This is a different matter from excessive cytokine production, which has emerged as an important factor in the pathogenesis of severe malaria. It has been estimated that life-threatening complications arise in about 1% of *P. falciparum* infections in Gambian children (Greenwood et al, 1987). If this figure sounds small it should be remembered that many African children are repeatedly infected with *P. falciparum*, resulting in over a million childhood deaths on that continent each year. Cerebral malaria and severe malaria anaemia are responsible for most of these deaths. Other complications of falciparum malaria include circulatory collapse, jaundice, renal failure, pulmonary oedema and disseminated intravascular coagulation, but intriguingly these are rarely seen in African children (Warrell et al, 1990). The latter complications resemble those of endotoxic shock, and this led to the early suggestion that severe bacterial sepsis and severe malaria might share common pathological mechanisms (Clark, 1978). TNF is now known to be a critical mediator of endotoxic shock (Beutler and Cerami, 1989), so it is reasonable to infer that it is at least partly responsible for the corresponding features of severe malaria. However falciparum malaria is quite different from other severe infections in its two most important complications, cerebral malaria and profound anaemia. Excessive cytokine production appears to be involved in both of these pathological processes.

The defining feature of cerebral malaria is unrousable coma, often associated with convulsions. In children this is sometimes accompanied by profound hypoglycaemia, but the coma of true cerebral malaria persists after hypoglycaemia is corrected. Case fatality rates in hospital are typically 10–15%. Gross neurological sequelae are observed in around 10% of children who survive, but appear to be much less common in adults

(Brewster et al, 1990). Clinically the most remarkable aspect of cerebral malaria in African children is that most deaths occur within 24 hours of onset, while most survivors make a full recovery within 4 or 5 days. The transience of the clinical symptoms and the general absence of cerebral oedema distinguish cerebral malaria from other forms of infectious encephalopathy. Histopathologically, the most striking finding is dense parasite sequestration in small cerebral blood vessels (MacPherson et al, 1985; Berendt et al, 1994).

Three lines of evidence, when taken together, strongly indicate that excessive TNF production is a causal factor in the pathogenesis of cerebral malaria. First, cerebral malaria is associated with high TNF levels (Grau et al, 1989; Kern et al, 1989), especially when children who die or develop neurological sequelae are compared with children with uncomplicated malaria fever (Kwiatkowski et al, 1990). Second, experimental studies have revealed a number of ways in which TNF could act to exacerbate the problem of parasite sequestration in cerebral blood vessels. Studies of *P. berghei* ANKA infection in CBA-Ca mice (Grau et al, 1987, 1991) led to the recognition that TNF can promote sequestration by upregulating specific endothelial adhesion molecules, such as intercellular adhesion molecule-1 and E-selectin (ELAM-1), which bind to molecules expressed on the surface of parasitized erythrocytes (Berendt et al, 1989, 1992; Ockenhouse et al, 1992). Apart from its role in promoting sequestration, TNF generated within cerebral blood vessels may have damaging effects on the surrounding brain. An intriguing suggestion, which might explain the transience of the coma, is that locally high TNF concentrations may stimulate cerebral endothelium to release huge amounts of nitric oxide, thus interfering with neurotransmission in the surrounding brain (Clark et al, 1991). The third line of evidence, which argues strongly for a causal relationship, is that genetic variation within the TNF promoter region is associated with susceptibility to cerebral malaria (McGuire et al, 1994). This result is discussed in more detail in the next section.

Experimental data indicate that TNF may also be relevant to severe malarial anaemia. In African children this is usually defined as a haemoglobin level of less 5 g/dl, this being the point at which heart failure becomes a significant risk even in children who have adapted to nutritional anaemia. Multiple factors contribute to its pathogenesis. The process of parasite replication, which destroys erythrocytes, can severely deplete haemoglobin levels if parasitaemia is very high or if the infection is prolonged. However, this is clearly only part of the story, and other important pathogenic elements include depression of erythrocyte production and phagocytosis of intact erythrocytes (Phillips et al, 1986). TNF can suppress erythropoiesis and promote erythrophagocytosis, and has been observed to do both in murine malaria (Clark and Chaudhri, 1988; Miller et al, 1989). In transgenic mice who constitutively overexpress TNF, malaria infections are controlled at a lower level of parasite density but they are also more likely to develop anaemia (Taverne et al, 1994). These mice exhibit increased erythrophagocytosis, which presumably contributes both to the anaemia and to the control of parasitaemia, an excellent example of the protective versus pathological effects of cytokine production in malaria. Clinical observation on cytokines and malaria anaemia are scanty, but it is known that many severe cases are associated with a long duration of symptoms, low parasitaemia and mild or absent fever (Abdalla et al, 1980) and we have found that TNF levels in this group are low when compared to levels in acute malaria fever or cerebral malaria (unpublished data). This might seem to imply low production but TNF has a short plasma half-life and this finding is also consistent with chronic overproduction. It favours the idea that malarial anaemia is exacerbated by sustained TNF production due to chronic infection, as distinct from the acutely high levels that predispose to cerebral malaria.

Though TNF is strongly implicated in the pathogenesis of cerebral malaria and circumstantially implicated in severe malarial anaemia, in both cases it probably plays a contributory rather than a primary role. The best evidence for this is the observation that plasma TNF levels are as high in uncomplicated vivax malaria as in cerebral malaria (Karunaweera et al, 1992b). Of course plasma levels may be a misleading indicator of TNF production rates, because of its short half-life, and it is important to consider how TNF may be synergizing with other cytokines (Rockett et al, 1993). However, the most important difference between vivax and falciparum malaria is that the two parasite species behave quite differently within the human host, and thus provide different opportunities for cytokine-induced pathology. In *P. falciparum* infection, parasite density is typically around 100-fold higher than in *P. vivax* infection (Kitchen, 1949), and schizonts of this species sequester in post-capillary venules. These elements of parasite behaviour are almost certainly the fundamental risk factors for severe anaemia and cerebral malaria, and it is contributory circumstances such as the dynamics of cytokine production that determine whether or not these complications actually occur.

BIOLOGICAL VARIATION

Over the past few years, several studies have indicated that humans differ in the amount of TNF that they produce in response to common stimuli such as bacterial lipopolysaccharide (LPS), and that these individual differences are stable over time. The question is whether such differences in TNF production are genetic and, if so, what are the variable gene(s) in question. It is not a trivial question because multiple genes might well be involved, from the LPS receptor through to the genes that control protein export, but the most obvious place to start to look was close to the TNF gene itself. Fortunately the TNF gene has an extremely convenient chromosomal location when it comes to addressing this type of question. It lies within the class III region of the major histocompatibility complex (MHC), which in humans is on chromosome 6; in other words it is sandwiched between the highly polymorphic genes of the MHC class I genes (e.g. HLA-B) and class

II (e.g. HLA-DR: Carroll et al, 1987; Dunham et al, 1987). The first evidence for genetic variation in TNF responsiveness was that individual differences in TNF production appeared to be linked to HLA type and other polymorphic markers that are close to the TNF gene (Molvig et al, 1988; Jacob et al, 1990; Pociot et al, 1993). However, such findings are simply clues as to the general location of a variable genetic element that controls TNF production. A strong candidate for such an element lies within the TNF promoter region, i.e. the stretch of DNA that lies immediately 5′ of the transcriptional start site of the gene, this being crucial to the regulation of transcription. There is a biallelic polymorphism at −308 nucleotides relative to the transcriptional start site of TNF (Wilson et al, 1993), and there is preliminary evidence that single base changes at or adjacent to this locus markedly affect transcriptional activity when linked to reporter constructs in B cells (Wilson et al, 1994). TNF transcription is higher for the less common allele, designated TNF2, and in The Gambia this has a gene frequency of around 0.16 (meaning that around 30% of Gambians carry at least one copy of the gene). It has been observed in a case–control study that Gambian children who are homozygous for the TNF2 allele have a relative risk of 4 for cerebral malaria, and of 7 for death or severe neurological sequelae due to cerebral malaria (McGuire et al, 1994). Importantly, this association with cerebral malaria was independent of variation in neighbouring HLA alleles, and it is consistent with the previous finding that circulating TNF levels are abnormally elevated in Gambian children with cerebral malaria, and highest in those who die or develop neurological sequelae (Kwiatkowski et al, 1990). The implication is that TNF2 homozygotes are predisposed to produce too much TNF and thereby run an increased risk of developing cerebral malaria. If this is so, then the high frequency of the TNF2 allele in The Gambia presumably reflects some biological advantage to the heterozygotes, perhaps in relation to malaria or some other life-threatening infection.

The parasite also varies. Wide differences have been observed in the TNF-inducing activity of different strains of *P. falciparum*. In experiments where human mononuclear cells are stimulated by whole parasite lysates in vitro, the amount of TNF induced by two parasite lines can differ by well over ten-fold (Allan et al, 1993). Some of these differences are due to the experimental variation that inevitably occurs in bioassays of this sort, but in replicated experiments it is clear that certain parasite lines consistently elicit a much larger TNF response than others. A question of considerable interest is whether TNF-inducing activity is linked to other polymorphisms such as the cytoadherence phenotype (Roberts et al, 1992). Within one parasite line an association was noted with rosetting ability (Allan et al, 1993), and other workers have suggested a link to expression of ring-infected erythrocyte surface antigen expression (Picot et al, 1993). However, these are not strong links and the molecular basis of variation in the TNF-inducing phenotype remains unknown, though it is tempting to speculate that it is due to genetic differences in the structure or level of expression of the major toxin. Preliminary attempts have been made to look for an association between disease severity and TNF-inducing phenotype.

When wild isolates were compared in vitro, it was observed that those from cerebral malaria patients tended to stimulate higher levels of TNF production than those from patients with uncomplicated malaria fever, but there was considerable overlap and the difference between the two groups was far from conclusive (Allan et al, 1995). However, there are various technical obstacles in this sort of clinical investigation. For example, experiments using cloned lines show that considerable heterogeneity can exist within a single infecting strain of parasite, and it is not clear whether parasites sampled from peripheral blood provide an accurate reflection of the subpopulation of parasites that are sequestered in the brain. Thus, it may be difficult to prove or refute the hypothesis that high TNF-inducing strains predispose to cerebral malaria. For the present, it is intriguing simply to note that such a wide degree of strain variation exists, given the part played by TNF in both protection and pathology.

Is this host and parasite polymorphism accidental? Here it has been argued that the TNF response provides a forms of innate immunity that regulates the density of malaria parasites within the host, but it does not eradicate the infection. It benefits the host but it also enhances the capacity of the host to act as a reservoir of infection. If this is an example of coevolutionary pragmatism on the part of parasite and host, then it is in the evolutionary interest of both parties to achieve an optimal level of TNF response with minimal risk of life-threatening pathology. But TNF is also important in other serious infections (tuberculosis is just one example) and the level of response that is optimal for one infection may be deleterious for another. Perhaps the polymorphisms described above represent the end result of host and parasite populations adapting to this evolutionary conundrum.

SUMMARY

Over the past decade it has emerged that parasite growth is inhibited at febrile temperatures, and that this is just part of a package of anti-parasitic mechanisms that are mediated through cytokines released by the host during fever paroxysms. This has led to the idea that fever, and the cytokine response with which it is associated, play an important role in the regulation of parasite density within the human host. At the same time it has become apparent that TNF and related host responses can be lethal in excess. Recent findings indicate that humans exhibit considerable genetic diversity in their levels of cytokine responsiveness, and that the sporadic occurrence of cerebral malaria and other life-threatening complications can be partly explained by individual differences in the cytokine response to infection. This illustrates the evolutionary need to balance the risk of cytokine-induced pathology against the benefits of this form of host defence. The aim of this chapter is to describe what is known about the host–parasite interaction that is clinically expressed as malaria fever, and to illustrate its relevance to the biology of infectious disease in general.

REFERENCES

Abdalla S, Weatherall DJ, Wickramasinghe SN & Hughes M (1980) The anaemia of *P. falciparum* malaria. *British Journal of Haematology* **46:** 171–183.

Allan RJ, Rowe A & Kwiatkowski D (1993) *Plasmodium falciparum* varies in its ability to induce tumor necrosis factor. *Infection and Immunity* **61:** 4772–4776.

Allan RJ, Beattie P, Bate CAW et al (1995) Strain variation in TNF induction by parasites from children with acute falciparum malaria. *Infection and Immunity* **63:** 1173–1175.

Allison AC & Eugui EM (1982) A radical interpretation of immunity to malaria parasites. *Lancet* **ii:** 1431–1433.

Bate CAW & Kwiatkowski D (1994a) A monoclonal antibody that recognises phosphatidylinositol inhibits induction of TNF alpha by different strains of *Plasmodium falciparum*. *Infection and Immunity* **62:** 5261–5266.

Bate CAW & Kwiatkowski D (1994b) Stimulators of tumour necrosis factor production released by damaged erythrocytes. *Immunology* **63:** 256–261.

Bate CAW, Taverne J & Playfair JHL (1988) Malarial parasites induce TNF production by macrophages. *Immunology* **64:** 227–231.

Bate CAW, Taverne J, Roman E et al (1991) TNF induction by malaria exoantigens depends on phospholipid. *Immunology* **75:** 129–135.

Bate CAW, Taverne J, Bootsma HZ et al (1992a) Antibodies against phosphatidylinositol and inositol monophosphate specifically inhibit TNF production by malaria exoantigens. *Immunology* **76:** 31–35.

Bate CAW, Taverne J, Karunaweera ND et al (1992b) Serological relationship of TNF-inducing exoantigens of *P. falciparum* and *P. vivax*. *Infection and Immunity* **60:** 1241–1243.

Bate CAW, Taverne J & Playfair JHL (1992c) Detoxified exoantigens and phosphatidylinositol derivatives inhibit tumor necrosis factor production by malaria exoantigens. *Infection and Immunity* **60:** 1894–1901.

Berendt AR, Simmons DL, Tansey J et al (1989) Intercellular adhesion molecule-1 is an endothelial cell adhesion receptor for *Plasmodium falciparum*. *Nature* **341:** 57–59.

Berendt AR, McDowall A, Craig AG et al (1992) The binding site of ICAM-1 for *Plasmodium falciparum*-infected erythrocytes overlaps, but is distinct from, the LFA-1 binding site. *Cell* **68:** 71–81.

Berendt AR, Turner G & Newbold CI (1994) Cerebral malaria: the sequestration hypothesis. *Parasitology Today* **10:** 412–414.

Beutler B & Cerami A (1989) The biology of cachectin/TNF—a primary mediator of the host response. *Annual Review of Immunology* **7:** 625–655.

Braun-Breton C, Rosenberry TL & Pereira da Silva L (1988) Induction of the proteolytic activity of a membrane protein in *Plasmodium falciparum* by phosphatidylinositol-specific phospholipase C. *Nature* **332:** 457–459.

Brewster DR, Kwiatkowski D & White NJ (1990) Neurological sequelae of cerebral malaria in children. *Lancet* **336:** 1039–1043.

Brown WH (1912) Malarial pigment (hematin) as a factor in the production of the malarial paroxysm. *Journal of Experimental Medicine* **15:** 579–597.

Butcher GA, Garland T, Ajdukiewicz AB & Clark IA (1990) Serum tumor necrosis factor associated with malaria in patients in the Solomon Islands. *Transactions of the Royal Society of Tropical Medicine and Hygiene* **84:** 658–661.

Cannon JG, van der Meer JWM, Kwiatkowski D et al (1988) Interleukin-1 beta in human plasma: optimization of blood collection, plasma extraction and radioimmunoassay methods. *Lymphokine Research* **7:** 457–467.

Carroll MC, Katzman P, Alicot EM et al (1987) Linkage map of the human major histocompatibility complex including the tumor necrosis factor genes. *Proceedings of the National Academy of Sciences of the USA* **84:** 8535–8539.

Clark IA (1978) Does endotoxin cause both the disease and parasite death in acute malaria and babesiosis? *Lancet* **ii:** 75–77.

Clark IA & Chaudhri G (1988) Tumour necrosis factor may contribute to the anaemia of malaria by causing dyserythropoesis and erythrophagocytosis. *British Journal of Haematology* **70:** 99–103.

Clark IA & Hunt NH (1983) Evidence for reactive oxygen intermediates causing hemolysis and parasite death in malaria. *Infection and Immunity* **39:** 1–6.

Clark IA, Virizelier J-L, Carswell EA & Wood PR (1981) Possible importance of macrophage-derived mediators in acute malaria. *Infection and Immunity* 32: 1058–1066.

Clark IA, Butcher GA, Buffinton GD et al (1987a) Toxicity of certain products of lipid peroxidation to the human malaria parasite *Plasmodium falciparum*. *Biochemical Pharmacology* 36: 543–546.

Clark IA, Hunt NH, Butcher GA & Cowden WB (1987b) Inhibition of murine malaria (*Plasmodium chabaudi*) in vivo by recombinant interferon-gamma or tumor necrosis factor, and its enhancement by butylated hydroxyanisole. *Journal of Immunology* 139: 3493–3496.

Clark IA, Rockett KA & Cowden WB (1991) Proposed link between cytokines, nitric oxide, and human cerebral malaria. *Parasitology Today* 7: 205–207.

Clark IA, Gray KM, Rockett EJ et al (1992) Increased lymphotoxin in human malarial serum, and the ability of this cytokine to increase plasma interleukin-6 and cause hypoglycaemia in mice: implications for malarial pathology. *Transactions of the Royal Society of Tropical Medicine and Hygiene* 86: 602–607.

Cranston WI (1966) Temperature regulation. *British Medical Journal* ii: 69–75.

Dinarello CA (1987) Interleukins, tumor necrosis factors (cachectin), and interferons as endogenous pyrogens and mediators of fever. *Lymphokines* 14: 1–31.

Dinarello CA (1991) Interleukin-1 and interleukin-1 antagonism. *Blood* 77: 1627–1652.

Dinarello CA & Cannon JG (1993) Cytokine measurements in septic shock. *Annals of Internal Medicine* 1198: 853–854.

Dinarello CA, Cannon JG, Wolff SM et al (1986) Tumor necrosis factor (cachectin) is an endogenous pyrogen and induces production of interleukin-1. *Journal of Experimental Medicine* 163: 1433–1450.

Dockrell HM & Playfair JHL (1983) Killing of blood-stage malaria parasites by hydrogen peroxide. *Infection and Immunity* 39: 456–459.

Dockrell HM & Playfair JHL (1984) Killing of *Plasmodium yoelii* by enzyme-induced products of the oxidative burst. *Infection & Immunity* 43: 451–456.

Dunham I, Sargent CA, Trowsdale J & Campbell RD (1987) Molecular mapping of the human major histocompatibility complex by pulsed-field gel electrophoresis. *Proceedings of the National Academy of Sciences of the USA* 84: 7237–7241.

Felton SC, Prior RB, Spagna VA & Kreier JP (1980) Evaluation of *Plasmodium berghei* for endotoxin by the *Limulus* lysate assay. *Journal of Parasitology* 66: 846–847.

Ferguson MAJ (1994) What can GPI do for you? *Parasitology Today* 11: 48–52.

Gerold P, Dieckmann-Schuppert A & Schwarz RT (1993) Glycosylphosphatidylinositols synthesized by asexual erythrocytic stages of the malarial parasite, *Plasmodium falciparum*. Candidates for plasmodial glycosylphosphatidylinositol membrane anchor precursors and pathogenicity factors. *Journal of Biological Chemistry* 269: 2597–2606.

Glew RH & Levin J (1975) Failure to demonstrate circulating endotoxin in malaria. *Proceedings of the Society of Experimental Biology and Medicine* 148: 508–510.

Golgi C (1889) Sul ciclo evolutio dei parassiti malarici nella febbre terzana: diagnosi differenziale tra i parassiti endoglobulari malarici della terzana e quelli della quartana. *Archivo per le Scienza Mediche* 13: 173–196. (On the cycle of development of malarial parasites in tertian fever: differential diagnosis between the intracellular malarial parasites of tertian and quartan fever. Extracts reprinted in Kean BH, Mott KE & Russell AJ (eds) *Tropical Medicine and Parasitology: Classic Investigations*. vol. 1, pp 26–35. Ithaca, 1978: Cornell University Press.

Grau GE, Fajardo LF, Piguet P-F et al (1987) Tumor necrosis factor (cachectin) as an essential mediator in murine cerebral malaria. *Science* 237: 1210–1212.

Grau GE, Taylor TE, Molyneux ME et al (1989) Tumor necrosis factor and disease severity in children with falciparum malaria. *New England Journal of Medicine* 320: 1586–1591.

Grau GE, Pointaire P, Piguet P-F et al (1991) Late administration of monoclonal antibody to leucocyte function-antigen 1 abrogates incipient murine cerebral malaria. *European Journal of Immunology* 21: 2265–2267.

Greenwood BM, Evans-Jones LG & Stratton D (1975) Failure to detect endotoxin in serum of children with malaria. *Lancet* ii: 874–875.

Greenwood BM, Bradley AK, Greenwood AM et al (1987) Mortality and morbidity from malaria among children in a rural area of The Gambia, West Africa. *Transactions of the Royal Society of Tropical Medicine and Hygiene* 81: 478–486.

Haldar K, Ferguson MAJ & Cross GAM (1985) Acylation of a *Plasmodium falciparum* merozoite surface antigen via *sn*-1,2-diacyl glycerol. *Journal of Biological Chemistry* 260: 4969–4974.

Jacob CO, Fronek Z, Lewis GD et al (1990) Heritable major histocompatibility complex class II-associated differences in production of tumor necrosis factor α: relevance to genetic predisposition to systemic lupus erythematosus. *Proceedings of the National Academy of Sciences of the USA* **87**: 1233–1237.

Jakobsen PH, Baek L & Jepsen S (1988) Demonstration of soluble *Plasmodium falciparum* antigens reactive with *Limulus* amoebocyte lysate and polymixin B. *Parasite Immunology* **10**: 593–606.

Jakobsen PH, Hviid L, Theander TG et al (1991) Isolation and characterization of a soluble antigen complex of *Plasmodium falciparum* with pyrogenic properties. *Acta Pathologica Microbiologica et Immunologica Scandinavica* **99**: 21–29.

Jakobsen PH, Moon R, Ridley RG et al (1993) Tumour necrosis factor and interleukin-6 production induced by components associated with merozoite proteins of *Plasmodium falciparum*. *Parasite Immunology* **15**: 229–237.

Jensen JB, van de Waa JA & Karadsheh AJ (1987) Tumor necrosis factor does not induce *Plasmodium falciparum* crisis forms. *Infection and Immunity* **55**: 1722–1724.

Karunaweera ND, Carter R, Grau GE et al (1992a) Tumour necrosis factor-dependent parasite-killing effects during paroxysms in non-immune *Plasmodium vivax* malaria patients. *Clinical and Experimental Immunology* **88**: 499–505.

Karunaweera ND, Grau GE, Gamage P et al (1992b) Dynamics of fever and serum levels of tumor necrosis factor are closely associated during clinical paroxysms in *Plasmodium vivax* malaria. *Proceedings of the National Academy of Sciences of the USA* **89**: 3200–3203.

Kern P, Hemmer CJ, van Damme J et al (1989) Elevated tumor necrosis factor alpha and interleukin-6 serum levels as markers for complicated *Plasmodium falciparum* malaria. *American Journal of Medicine* **57**: 139–143.

Kitchen SF (1949) Chapters on symptomatology, falciparum malaria, quartan malaria, and vivax malaria. In Boyd MF (ed.) *Malariology*, vol. 2, pp 966–1045. Philadelphia: WB Saunders.

Kluger MJ (1979) *Fever: Its Biology, Evolution and Function*. Princeton, NJ: Princeton University Press.

Kluger MJ (1991) Fever: role of pyrogens and cryogens. *Physiological Reviews* **71**: 93–127.

Kumaratilake LM, Ferrante A & Rzepczyk C (1991) The role of T lymphocytes in immunity to *Plasmodium falciparum*. Enhancement of neutrophil-mediated parasite killing by lymphotoxin and IFN-gamma: comparison with tumour necrosis factor effects. *Journal of Immunology* **146**: 762–767.

Kwiatkowski D (1989) Febrile temperatures can synchronise the growth of *Plasmodium falciparum* in vitro. *Journal of Experimental Medicine* **169**: 357–361.

Kwiatkowski D (1991) Cytokines and anti-disease immunity to malaria. *Research in Immunology* **142**: 707–712.

Kwiatkowski D & Greenwood BM (1989) Why is malaria fever periodic? *Parasitology Today* **5**: 264–266.

Kwiatkowski D & Nowak M (1991) Periodic and chaotic host–parasite interactions in human malaria. *Proceedings of the National Academy of Sciences of the USA* **88**: 5111–5113.

Kwiatkowski D, Cannon JG, Manogue KR et al (1989) Tumour necrosis factor production in falciparum malaria and its association with schizont rupture. *Clinical and Experimental Immunology* **77**: 361–366.

Kwiatkowski D, Hill AVS, Sambou I et al (1990) TNF concentration in fatal cerebral, non-fatal cerebral, and uncomplicated *Plasmodium falciparum* malaria. *Lancet* **336**: 1201–1204.

Kwiatkowski D, Molyneux ME, Stephens S et al (1993) Anti-TNF therapy inhibits fever in cerebral malaria. *Quarterly Journal of Medicine* **86**: 91–98.

MacGregor RR, Sheagren JN & Wolff SM (1969) Endotoxin-induced modification of *Plasmodium berghei* infection in mice. *Journal of Immunology* **102**: 131–139.

MacPherson GG, Warrell MJ, White NJ et al (1985) Human cerebral malaria: a quantitative ultrastructural analysis of parasitized erythrocyte sequestration. *American Journal of Pathology* **119**: 385–401.

Martin LK, Einheber A, Sadun EH & Wren RE (1967) Effect of bacterial endotoxin on the course of *Plasmodium berghei* infection. *Experimental Parasitology* **20**: 186–199.

McGuire W, Hill AVS, Allsopp CEM et al (1994) Variation in the TNF-α promoter region is associated with susceptibility to cerebral malaria. *Nature* **371**: 508–511.

Meding SJ & Langhorne J (1991) CD4+ T cells and B cells are necessary for the transfer of protective immunity to *Plasmodium chabaudi chabaudi*. *European Journal of Immunology* **21**: 1433–1438.

Miller KL et al (1989) Tumor necrosis factor-alpha and the anemia associated with murine malaria. *Infection and Immunity* **57**: 1542–1546.

Molvig J, Baek L, Christensen P et al (1988) Endotoxin-stimulated human monocyte secretion of interleukin 1, tumor necrosis factor alpha, and prostaglandin E_2 shows stable interindividual differences. *Scandinavian Journal of Immunology* **27**: 705–716.

Molyneux ME, Taylor TE, Wirima JJ & Grau GE (1991) Tumour necrosis factor, interleukin-1, and malaria. *Lancet* **337**: 1098.

Morrison DB & Anderson WAD (1942) On the role of parasite pigment in the malaria paroxysm. *Public Health Reports* **57**: 161–174.

Neifer S, Kremsner PG & Bienzle U (1989) Application of anti-TNF to *Plasmodium vinckei*-infected mice is followed by an increase of parasitaemia. *Acta Tropica* **46**: 273–275.

Nnalue NA & Friedman MJ (1988) Evidence for a neutrophil-mediated protective response in malaria. *Parasite Immunology* **10**: 47–58.

Ockenhouse CF & Shear HL (1984) Oxidative killing of the intraerythrocytic malaria parasite *Plasmodium yoelii* by activated macrophages. *Journal of Immunology* **132**: 424–431.

Ockenhouse CF, Tegoshi T, Maeno Y et al (1992) Human vascular endothelial cell adhesion receptors for *Plasmodium falciparum*-infected erythrocytes: roles for endothelial leukocyte adhesion molecule 1 and vascular cell adhesion molecule 1. *Journal of Experimental Medicine* **176**: 1183–1189.

Phillips RE, Looarewusan S (1986) The importance of anaemia in cerebral malaria and uncomplicated falciparum malaria: role of complications, dyserythropoiesis and iron sequestration. *Quarterly Journal of Medicine* **58**: 305–323.

Pichyangkul S, Saengkrai P & Webster HK (1994) *Plasmodium falciparum* pigment induces monocytes to release high levels of tumor necrosis factor alpha and interleukin 1-beta. *American Journal of Tropical Medicine and Hygiene* **51**: 430–435.

Picot S, Peyron F, Deloron P et al (1993) Ring-infected erythrocyte surface antigen (Pf155/RESA) induces tumor necrosis factor-alpha production. *Clinical and Experimental Immunology* **93**: 184–188.

Playfair JHL, Taverne J & Matthews N (1984) What is tumour necrosis factor really for? *Immunology Today* **5**: 165–166.

Pociot F, Briant L, Jongeneel CV et al (1993) Association of tumor necrosis factor (TNF) and class II major histocompatibility complex alleles with the secretion of TNF-α and TNF-β by human mononuclear cells: a possible link to insulin-dependent diabetes mellitus. *European Journal of Immunology* **23**: 224–231.

Roberts DJ, Craig AG, Berendt AR et al (1992) Rapid switching to multiple antigenic and adhesive phenotypes in malaria. *Nature* **357**: 689–692.

Roberts NJ (1991) Impact of temperature elevation on immunologic defenses. *Reviews of Infectious Diseases* **13**: 462–472.

Rockett KA, Awburn MM, Cowden WB & Clark IA (1991) Killing of *Plasmodium falciparum* in vitro by nitric oxide derivatives. *Infection and Immunity* **59**: 3280–3283.

Rockett KA, Awburn MM, Aggarwal BB et al (1992) In vivo induction of nitrite and nitate by tumor necrosis factor, lymphotoxin, and interleukin-1 implies a role for nitric oxide in cytokine-induced malarial cell-mediated immunity and pathology. *Infection and Immunity* **60**: 3725–3730.

Rockett KA, Awburn MM, Rockett EJ & Clark IA (1993) TNF and IL-1 synergy in the context of malarial pathology. *American Journal of Tropical Medicine and Hygiene* **50**: 735–742.

Ross R (1911) *The Prevention of Malaria*. 2nd edn. London: John Murray.

Schofield L & Hackett F (1993) Signal transduction in host cells by a glycosylphosphatidylinositol toxin of malaria parasites. *Journal of Experimental Medicine* **177**: 145–153.

Scuderi P, Sterling KE, Lam KS et al (1986) Raised serum levels of tumour necrosis factor in parasitic infections. *Lancet* **ii**: 1364–1365.

Shaffer N, Grau GE, Hedberg K et al (1991) Tumor necrosis factor and severe malaria. *Journal of Infectious Diseases* **163**: 96–101.

Slater AF, Swiggard WJ, Orton BR et al (1991) An iron-carboxylate bond links the heme units of malaria pigment. *Proceedings of the National Academy of Sciences of the USA* **88**: 325–329.

Smythe JA, Coppel RL, Brown GA et al (1988) Identification of two integral membrane proteins of *Plasmodium falciparum*. *Proceedings of the National Academy of Sciences of the USA* **85**: 5195–5199.

Stocker R, Hunt NH, Buffinton GD et al (1985) Oxidative stress and protective mechanisms in erythrocytes in relation to *Plasmodium vinckei* load. *Proceedings of the National Academy of*

Taverne J, Tavernier J, Fiers W & Playfair JHL (1987) Recombinant tumour necrosis factor inhibits malaria parasites *in vivo* but not *in vitro*. *Clinical Experimental Immunology* **67**: 1–4.

Taverne J, Bate CAW, Kwiatkowski D et al (1990) Two soluble antigens of *Plasmodium falciparum* induce tumor necrosis factor release from macrophages. *Infection and Immunity* **58**: 2923–2928.

Taverne J, Sheikh N, de Souza JB et al (1994) Anaemia and resistance to malaria in transgenic mice expressing human tumour necrosis factor. *Immunology* **82**: 397–403.

Taylor-Robinson AW, Phillips RS et al (1993) The role of T_H1 and T_H2 cells in a rodent malaria infection. *Science* **260**: 1931–1934.

Tubbs H (1980) Endotoxin in human and murine malaria. *Transactions of the Royal Society of Tropical Medicine and Hygiene* **74**: 121–123.

Warrell DA, Molyneux ME & Beales P (1990) Severe and complicated malaria, 2nd edn. *Transactions of the Royal Society of Tropical Medicine and Hygiene* **84** (supplement 2): 1–65.

Wilson AG, de Vries N, Pociot F et al (1993) An allelic polymorphism within the human tumor necrosis factor alpha promoter region is strongly associated with HLA A1, B8 and DR3 alleles. *Journal of Experimental Medicine* **177**: 557–560.

Wilson AG, Symons JA, McDowell TL et al (1994) Effects of a tumour necrosis factor (TNF-α) promoter base transition on transcriptional activity. *British Journal of Rheumatology* **33** (supplement 10): 89.

Wozencraft AO, Dockrell HM, Taverne J et al (1984) Killing of human malaria parasites by macrophage secretory products. *Infection and Immunity* **43**: 664–669.

10

Strategies towards the design of a synthetic subunit malaria vaccine

ROBERTO AMADOR
MAURICIO ROJAS
MARIO A. POSADA
ALBERTO MORENO
MANUEL E. PATARROYO

Malaria represents by far the most important parasitic disease in man. The World Health Organization (WHO) has calculated that the number of infected people increased at the rate of 5% annually (Kolberg, 1994). The enthusiasm of the 1950s for possible malaria control has been replaced by the pessimism of the 1980s and 1990s due to the failure of insecticides and chemotherapy to eliminate the insect vectors or parasites. New strategies have been proposed such as vector control by gene manipulation and immunoprophylaxis by vaccines. The plasticity of the vector, and the diverse stages within the parasite life cycle raise major obstacles to vaccine design (Aldhous, 1994).

The complexity of the life cycle of the parasite is but one factor that has hindered the development of an effective vaccine against *Plasmodium falciparum*. Vaccines must be targeted at the different stages and contain both B and T cell epitopes. The main objective of this approach is to develop protective immunity and then to use natural exposure as a means of boosting immunity. This is particularly important in areas of high endemicity where the most susceptible are children under 5 years of age.

Considerable research has been carried out on sporozoite and blood stage antigens, several of which have been considered as promising vaccine candidates, but comparatively few human trials have been performed. The criteria for the selection of antigens, as vaccine components, have been based on the ability to induce humoral or cellular specific immunity or the property of the candidates to induce protection to experimental challenge in animal models (Pasloke and Howard, 1994).

Our group began research on the immunology of malaria a decade ago. This research has led to the development of an inexpensive synthetic subunit vaccine that is currently undergoing major field trials worldwide. This subunit vaccine, SPf66, combining preerythrocytic and asexual blood stage antigens, has been the only one to undergo large-scale field trials to date. Recent reviews of studies dealing with the many problems encountered in malaria vaccine development can be found elsewhere (Nussenzweig and Nussenzweig, 1989; Lussow et al, 1990; Nussenzweig, 1990; Del Giudice, 1991; Esposito et al, 1991; Good, 1991; Good et al, 1992; Romero, 1992; Nussenzweig and Long, 1994). In this chapter we wish to discuss the approach that we have used for development and testing of the first generation of multiantigenic and multistage synthetic peptide malaria vaccines. We also emphasize the general problems to be considered for future subunit vaccines.

BACKGROUND

In areas highly endemic for malaria the target populations that receives the major benefits from the introduction of effective vaccines, are children under 5 years of age and pregnant women. The objective of immunization strategy is to induce clinical immunity in the susceptible population. Under normal conditions this type of protection is only achieved after a number of potentially serious, sometimes life-threatening, natural infections.

A number of conceptual problems need to be considered in the development of subunit malaria vaccines. For example, antibodies obtained from people living in malaria endemic areas are not always capable of inhibiting the invasion of merozoites into erythrocytes in in vitro assays, suggesting more complex mechanisms of naturally acquired protection (Marsh et al, 1989). This observation is consistent with the high degree of polymorphism of several antigens expressed on the malaria parasite or antigenic variation (De La Cruz et al, 1989; Kaslow et al, 1989; Shi et al, 1992). Neutralizing antibodies capable of inhibiting invasion need to be of high affinity. The design of vaccines must therefore consider the identification of conserved antigenic determinants able to induce protective antibodies, whatever their mode of action. For example, parasite organelles such as rhoptries and micronemes involved in the process of invasion are intracellular and therefore access of antibodies to these cryptic structures could limit their blocking effect (Holder, 1994).

The feasibility of developing effective malaria vaccines has been prompted by the successful immunization of susceptible hosts with irradiated sporozoites or whole merozoites (Reese et al, 1978; Clyde, 1990). However, this classical approach using whole cells or organisms is not achievable due to logistic problems related to the setting up of large scale culture systems for mass vaccination and the biohazard and risks of autoimmunity associated with the use of human material (i.e. red blood cells). Therefore, our current approach has focused on vaccines based on recombinant proteins or synthetic peptide chemistry.

Preerythrocytic vaccines are aimed at blocking the development of recently inoculated parasites. Considering the variability of the inoculum and the high rate of division within the hepatocyte, preerythrocytic vaccines need to substantially reduce the development of the liver stage parasites. Their effectiveness must be at a range well above 90% to prevent progression of the disease. Such a vaccine could theoretically prevent high levels of parasitaemia, which may be particularly important in people living in endemic areas.

Blood stage vaccines, whilst not necessarily eradicating all parasites, aim to decrease the level of parasitaemia and thus disease severity. Decrease in parasite multiplication should theoretically modify the mortality and severity of the disease. Even partial immunity to the asexual blood stage parasites could be useful, since disease severity is generally related to the level of parasitaemia (Greenwood et al, 1987). A vaccine directed against the asexual blood stages could delay or abrogate the development of life-threatening infection. Additional approaches include the development of an anti-disease vaccine that may not decrease parasite multiplication but could, for example, inhibit the adherence of infected red blood cells to endothelial cells (Ringwald et al, 1993) or decrease the production of toxic factors such as tumour necrosis factor (TNF) and nitric oxide (NO) released in response to a malaria toxin (Bate and Kwiatkowski, 1994a,b).

Another approach has been to develop sexual blood stage or trans-mission-blocking vaccines to impede the sexual reproduction of the parasite. These vaccines could destroy gametocytes, interfere with fertilization or prevent the development of the parasite within the mosquito. Such a vaccine would control the disease in communities rather than protect a given individual from disease.

DEVELOPMENT OF THE SYNTHETIC SPf66 COLOMBIAN MALARIA VACCINE

The rationale for a synthetic malaria subunit vaccine (SPf66) was based on the suggestion that multiple antigens were likely to be involved in the invasion of red blood cells. Several proteins were isolated from wild strains of *P. falciparum* on the basis that they were expressed on the merozoite surface (Patarroyo et al, 1987a). Further characterization of the proteins included determination of the N-terminal amino acid sequence and immunogenicity of the isolated proteins and peptides synthesized, based on the derived sequence of the proteins (Patarroyo et al, 1987b).

In the Colombian night monkey (*Aotus trivirgatus*) model, eight out of 40 different synthesized peptides induced immune responses that were partially protective. Monkeys immunized with a combination of two or three synthetic peptides coupled to bovine serum albumin (BSA) as carrier, developed high titres of antibodies reactive with native proteins present on *P. falciparum* merozoites. When challenged with infected red blood cells, three out of six monkeys immunized with a mixture of three peptides (83.1, 55.1 and 35.1), developed only low parasitaemia levels that peaked between days 10 and 15, significantly later than in the control groups, and went on to recover spontaneously. The remaining three animals did not develop parasitaemias. Using these data, a hybrid synthetic polymeric mol-ecule was designed. The rationale for the development of the SPf66 was based on the fact that in humans a safe and effective carrier protein would be difficult to achieve. The molecule consists of three epitopes based on amino acid sequences derived from three blood stage proteins (85, 55 and 35 kDa), intercalated by PNANP sequences derived from the immunodominant B cell epitope on the circumsporozoite protein of *P. falciparum*. The synthetic hybrid subunit vaccine, SPf66, was immunogenic and induced protective response in *Aotus* monkeys. This experiment has been repeated several times with larger groups of animals, showing similar results (Rodriguez et al, 1990).

Preclinical studies were completed using *Aotus* monkeys to test toxicity and safety. Pyrogenicity and sterility tests were performed for each batch of vaccine in rabbits. Immediately before, and eight days after, each immunization, the animals were bled for analysis of renal and hepatic function, blood count and blood chemistry. No statistically significant differences were found between groups immunized with the SPf66 vaccine and the control. Fifteen days after application of each dose, one animal from each group was sacrificed for anatomopathologic studies.

We routinely use the *Aotus* monkey model which remains the most suitable for simulating human *P. falciparum* infection (Special Programme for Research and Training in Tropical Diseases, 1988). These monkeys, unlike other animal models, are highly susceptible to malaria, and in them the disease is uniformly lethal unless treated or protected by vaccination. In addition, host factors, such as genetic restriction, have also influenced the immune response in an outbred *Aotus* population (Collins, 1992). Controversy over the use of monkeys for the development of malaria vaccines has been raised. The clinical course of the disease in non-human primates and the feasibility of controlling a second infection suggests biological constraints (Druilhe and Pérignon, 1994). Nevertheless, the importance of testing future vaccines in an animal model cannot be understated.

In order to assess local and systemic tolerability and immune response to the inoculated antigens in humans, 30 out of 109 volunteers from the Colombian Military were further examined. Thirteen individuals were finally selected for testing of the vaccine based on physical, clinical and psychological examination. The results of the Phase I clinical trial showed that the vaccine was well tolerated, with only minor local reactions being observed in a few cases. None of the volunteers presented with fever or showed significant changes in blood cell count, blood chemistry and urinalysis on days −1, 1, 3 and 5 after each immunization. Autoimmunity tests (rheumatoid factor, anti-nuclear antibodies, Coombs test and anti-myocardial fibre antibodies) were uniformly negative. The volunteers developed moderate anti-peptide responses, and all of them recognized the native proteins expressed on *P. falciparum* merozoites. Peripheral blood lymphocytes obtained from the volunteers were able to proliferate when tested in vitro with the synthetic polymer (Patarroyo et al, 1988).

The vaccinees were challenged by intravenous inoculation with 1×10^6 infected erythrocytes. During intravenous challenge, it was regarded as more important to use clinical, rather than parasitological parameters in order to ascertain when to treat patients. It was thus possible to follow up the volunteers for a longer time to document delay in disease progression. All the individuals were free to withdraw from the study whenever they chose to do so, as occurred with one of the individuals participating in the trials with the SPf66 vaccine. Of the five individuals immunized with the SPf66 vaccine, three were protected when challenged, one retired in mid-study, and one required drug treatment. The calculated efficacy of the vaccine for this early trial was 75% (Patarroyo et al, 1988).

According to WHO guidelines, the efficacy of any vaccine should then be assessed through natural exposure to the parasite under endemic conditions. For this study, 399 male volunteers, aged 18 to 21 in the Colombian Army, were chosen to participate in the study. Of these, 185 were vaccinated with the SPf66 hybrid polymer, and the remaining 214 served as controls. Different schedules of immunization were tested to establish the optimal regimen to be used in subsequent studies. These soldiers, who had little previous exposure to the parasite, were on patrolling missions within a wide endemic area on Colombia's southwest coastline. This area presents an annual parasitological index (API) of 12 (±2)%, with an incidence of 80–90% of *P. falciparum*.

Vaccinated volunteers were carefully monitored, and any who developed febrile symptoms were evacuated to the Tumaco Regional Military Health Center (RMHC) for clinical and laboratory tests. Blood smears of these individuals were read blindly and independently by the staff members of the Tumaco RMHC and the Servicio de Erradicación de la Malaria (SEM) in Tumaco. Both these results were reread by staff at the SEM's Central Laboratory in Bogotá to either confirm or refute the original diagnosis.

To evaluate the safety of the vaccine, a thorough clinical examination was performed on all volunteers during the first hour after each immunization, and then again at 24 and 48 hours. Blood chemistry and autoimmune tests were performed for each vaccinee 10 days after each immunization. No statistically significant differences were found when the vaccinated and control groups were compared. The efficacy of the vaccine was calculated as 82.3% against *P. falciparum* and 60.6% against *P. vivax*, although this was not a statistically significant trend (Rocha et al, 1992).

The IgG antibody production kinetics against the SPf66 vaccine were established in a parallel study. It was seen that these antibodies increased 15 to 30 days after the second and third immunization, clearly showing a boosting effect after the third dose. The antibodies were also shown to recognize native parasite proteins, as assessed by Western blots. However, the response was not the same in all individuals. Following the second immunization, a characteristic pattern of IgG response against the vaccine was observed using FAST-ELISA, whereby the vaccinees could be placed in three different groups. The first group, the high responders, presented antibody titres between 1 : 1600 and 1 : 25 600. A second group of intermediate responders showed antibody titres between 1 : 200 and 1 : 800, and a third group, the low responders, comprised all individuals in which antibody titres did not increase above 1 : 100 (Salcedo et al, 1991).

A further study showed a bimodal distribution of these antibodies in the vaccinated population, suggesting genetic control of the immune response to this protein. Consequently, HLA A, B, DR and DQ typing was performed on 105 vaccinees and 47 control individuals. The distribution of DR and DQ alleles of the high responders was similar to that of the control group. However, the population of HLA DR4 individuals within the low responder group (68%) was significantly higher when compared to the control group (36.2%) and the high responders (25%; Patarroyo et al, 1991). Using oligotyping methods after amplification of the DR4 B-1 exon, we proceeded to subtype 20 DR4 volunteers classified as either high, intermediate or low responders. No correlation was found between a specific DR4 subtype and the humoral immune response of the vaccinees (Murillo et al, 1992).

The results of the Tumaco A, B, C and D trials showed that the best immunization schedule for adults under these conditions consisted of three doses of the vaccine on days 0, 30 and 180, each containing 2 mg of the synthetic SPf66 polymer adsorbed onto 1 mg of alum hydroxide (Rocha et al, 1992).

A pilot study was performed in children aged 1–14 living in the endemic area of Tumaco, Colombia (Patarroyo et al, 1992). Of the 292 children receiving the three doses of the vaccine, 94.6% showed no adverse reaction. The remaining 12 children, presented slight local cutaneous reactions that did not persist at subsequent follow-up. No delayed adverse reactions were detected in the 62 children whom it was possible to evaluate 1 year after the first dose. Sera obtained from these children 20 days after the third immunization showed that 93.7% developed high titres to SPf66, ranging from 1 : 100 to 1 : 12 800, as determined by FAST-ELISA. In both studies, reactivity to native proteins, as assessed by Western blot, was high, especially to the 135, 115 and 83 kDa proteins. The results of these studies established beyond reasonable doubt, the safety and immunogenicity of the SPf66 vaccine.

Because initial field trials had been carried out with a small number of individuals living in non-endemic areas, the next field trial was carried out under more representative conditions, with individuals living in endemic areas. For this, the town of Majadas, in the state of Bolivar, in eastern Venezuela was chosen as the site for study by the research group, which comprised the Universidad Central de Venezuela and the Ministry of Health. This area is endemic for *P. falciparum*, with an API of 10% and a species infection rate of 25% for *P. falciparum*. Because of ethical considerations we decided not to exclude any individual over 11 years of age (except for pregnant women) who manifested a desire to receive the vaccine. Thus, 976 (27.6%) of the townspeople were immunized three times with SPf66, with 938 unvaccinated. The two groups were comparable. The aim of this study was to evaluate any change in the epidemiological characteristics of the vaccinated population when compared with the non-vaccinated population, and ascribe the difference to the effects of vaccination. To compare the incidence of malaria after vaccination between the vaccinated and the non-vaccinated groups adjusting for a dissimilar malaria risk at the baseline ratios were calculated for the incidence rate during the 12 month period subsequent to the third vaccine dose in relation to that observed during an equivalent calendar period of time just before vaccination. The after/before vaccination incidence ratio of each group was used to derive vaccine efficacy. The protective efficacy against *P. falciparum* for those receiving the complete series of three vaccination doses was calculated to be 55.1%. The protective effect of the vaccine against *P. vivax* was estimated as 41%, evidence that needs to be corroborated in future studies in *P. vivax* endemic areas (Amador et al, 1992).

Parallel to this study in Venezuela, our group in Colombia began a large trial with universal vaccination, randomized by localities and not by individuals, although pregnant women were excluded. For this, 9957 persons, all older than 1 year and inhabiting the Tumaco and Francisco Pizarro municipalities on the Colombian Southern Pacific coast, were administered three doses of the vaccine as defined previously. Of the vaccinees, 95.7% showed no adverse reactions to the vaccine. In the remaining 4.3%, local induration and erythema were the most frequent reactions. Among a randomly selected group of vaccinees, anti-SPf66 antibody titres were measured by ELISA, showing 55% with a titre above 1 : 1600.

As a result of a meeting in mid-1990 in Bogotá between our research group and a committee from the WHO, the necessity of initiating double-blind placebo trials under different malaria epidemiologic conditions was emphasized. These were initiated and are now being carried out in conjunction with other internationally recognized research groups in Colombia, Venezuela, Ecuador (Sampértegui et al, 1994), Brazil, Tanzania (Lopez et al, 1994; Teuscher et al, 1994), The Gambia and Thailand, involving from 500 to 3000 individuals. Variable efficacy is observed for any vaccine when applied to different populations, or even to different subgroups within a population, due to inherent differences in the immune status of the individuals, the pattern of transmission and intensity of the disease, the different parasite strains, etc. Therefore, it becomes essential to perform replicate trials under different epidemiological conditions.

Several aspects in the way these trials have been designed, which are a result of our previous experience in field trials, are worthy of mention.

Determination of the study population

Initial studies were selected according to criteria such as the behaviour of the disease during the past few years, malariometric indices (APIs for *P. falciparum* and *P. vivax*), which need to be sufficiently high for a statistical difference to be observed between vaccination and control groups, infrastructure of the locality, access, willingness of the community to participate in a trial, etc. It is known that in many remote areas in South America, malaria cases are grossly under-notified. For that reason, in several cases our group, or the research group conducting the particular field trial, chose the locality where the best records had been kept, in order to determine an adequate epidemiologic baseline. However, in some cases, even this information was not available, and in some cases we unavoidably had to base projection on incomplete data.

From leaders of the respective communities we determined the importance that town dwellers attributed to the disease. It must be noted that

Colombia is a leader in the WHO-sponsored Expanded Programs of Immunization (EPI), and thus vaccination is seen by most communities in a very positive light.

Once a locality was selected, the social workers, in close contact with the leaders of the community, achieved the participation of the entire community in the trial. The importance of these field workers and their interaction with the community cannot be overstated. These individuals went through extensive training in both malaria and the socioeconomic, cultural and anthropological characteristics of the population to be studied, and in many cases were inhabitants of these communities. Trial designs for the different localities were sometimes modified according to the recommendations of these individuals.

A census of the entire population was an important subsequent step, for it was the basis of the randomization procedure. The locality was dissected under demographic (racial) characteristics, occupation, malariometric and medical histories, physical examination, etc. Individuals with no previous history of allergy or debilitating disease and whose physical examination was normal were included in the study population. Pregnant women were excluded from the study. To establish whether a woman was pregnant, we performed blood or urine tests on every female aged 15 to 45. The tests were performed with blood samples and, if an ambiguous result was obtained, from a urine sample. Family heads and every person over 18 was asked to sign a consent form, accepting the fact this was a double-blind placebo-controlled trial, and that they could withdraw from the study whenever they chose to do so.

Individuals were assigned a code that greatly simplified the logistics of the study: the code consisted of a single letter, corresponding to the locality, followed by a two-digit number corresponding to the house number, and a last letter corresponding to the individual's place within the family. A house number was assigned by the malaria eradication/control institution of each country, and is widely used by most communities. This simplified the task of tracking down single individuals when necessary.

Randomization

Based on the census of the universal population, each individual was classified under four different groupings:

1. Locality.
2. Sex.
3. Age (1–4; 5–14; 15–45; 45 and older).
4. Occupation (farmers, fishermen, students, housewives, others).

Randomization was performed on the groups resulting in all possible combinations of these four categories. By keeping detailed records from each individual, the impact of some biases introduced into the study have been minimized.

Two different methods of randomizing the population were used. One method consisted of having a computer at the headquarters of the research group randomize the coded individuals, and the other was to perform the randomization procedure at the site of vaccination.

Vaccination

Prior to vaccination, the Ethics Committee designated by the Health Ministry of the respective country to monitor the field trial assigned letter codes to the vaccine and placebo vials, and these were then dispatched to the vaccination post.

Early on in the design of our first trials our group decided to use tetanus toxoid instead of plain aluminium hydroxide as placebo, although we were well aware of the possible biases introduced into the study by doing so. The main reason for this decision was an ethical one. We believed it was important for the individuals vaccinated with a placebo to receive at least some benefit by participating in this study. Besides, the physical aspect of both the tetanus toxoid and the SPf66 formulations, and the reactions they caused, were very similar. To minimize the possibility of the tetanus toxoid, an unspecific T-cell activator, interfering with the results of the trial, it was applied at the time of the first dose of the vaccine only. The other Latin American groups performing field trials with this vaccine have done likewise.

For logistical purposes, the vaccination post was divided into four different areas:

1. Registration site. It is at this point where randomization is controlled. The personnel at this site assign sequential letter codes to the members of each of the randomized groups in order of arrival, in the case of field randomization, or dictates the assigned code to the individual, in the case of randomization at headquarters, and checks that the requisites for vaccination have been completely fulfilled (signature on a consent form, complete medical and census data, etc.). The individual then passes on to the vaccination site.
2. Vaccination site. This site is unique for each vaccination post. The responsibility of vaccination with the correct letter-coded vial (as assigned by the registrar) rests with two people, in order to minimize the possibility of human error. After immunization, the vaccinee passes on to the third site within the vaccination post.
3. Observation site. The vaccinee remains for 30–45 minutes at this site. This provides a good opportunity to participate with the community in health education, and a place where questions regarding general health matters are answered. The site is staffed by two doctors.
4. Intensive care unit. Individuals who suffered any complications (local or systemic) during or after the 30 minute observation period were taken immediately to this site. The basic equipment in this unit consisted of an oxygen supply, respiratory support, intravenous liquids, drugs and even an ambulance when available. Intensivist doctors staffed this unit, and general practitioners who assisted in the site had received appropiate training for the purpose.

The importance of field workers was essential to guide individuals from site to site, and to reassure those who were anxious.

Post-vaccination

At 24 to 48 hours after each vaccination, a team of doctors performed a medical checkup on the vaccinees to ensure that none were suffering from delayed reactions. Apart from this, an independent Immediate Reaction Group (Grupo de Reacción Inmediata: GRI), made up of doctors belonging to governmental health institutions, heard and assessed complaints of any possible complication that might be attributed to the vaccine.

Epidemiologic monitoring

A field station was set up in each vaccination locality staffed by doctors, nurses and personnel from the governmental malaria control/eradication institutions from the respective countries. The facilities installed in each station included computers for the collection and primary analysis of statistical data, microscopes, vehicles, boats and communication systems. Both active and passive epidemiological monitoring were carried out for most trials. Active monitoring involved an intensive, house-to-house search by a group of doctors of any malaria cases. Passive monitoring was performed by people of the community, usually the leaders, who were trained in the reading of thick smears. This latter aspect turned out to be rather important, for it increased the coverage of the monitoring procedure, although it also reduced the power to detect the efficacy of the vaccine, for this intervention decreases the possibility of contracting malaria by reducing the number of gametocytes after early treatment. Diagnosis performed by these individuals was confirmed by an experienced field microscopist, and later by the central laboratories of the malaria eradication/control institutions of each country.

Defining 'clinical malaria' as an endpoint of the study in Latin America is easier than in Africa because subclinical parasitaemias are not often observed. For these reasons we defined malaria as a febrile episode, above 37.5°C, with the presence of peripheral blood parasitaemia. In contrast, an episode of clinical malaria in Tanzania was defined, for the trial, as measured fever (≥ 37.5°C) and parasite density $> 20\,000 / \mu l$. Contrary to what was done in Phase I trials, where constant monitoring of parasitaemias was performed for each and every individual, establishing the reduction of parasitaemias in a field trial is impossible both practically and ethically.

Phase III randomized, double-blind placebo-controlled clinical field trials, showed that the chemically synthesized SPf66 malaria vaccine was safe, non-toxic, immunogenic and protective against *P. falciparum* in semi-immune populations subjected to natural challenge, including children older than 1 year of age. The estimated protective efficacy of the vaccine was between 38.8% and 66.8%, being highest in children aged 1–4 years (77%: Valero et al, 1993). Studies carried out in Tanzania (Alonso et al, 1994) have confirmed that SPf66 is safe, immunogenic and reduces the risk of clinical malaria among children of the same age. The area chosen has an intense perennial *P. falciparum* transmission, where everyone receives more than 300 infective bites/year. The estimated vaccine efficacy was 31%. Finally, it should be noted for the record, that for trials performed outside of Colombia our laboratory has supplied the vaccine, assisted in the design of the trial, and was present in an observer status. In no case have we intervened in the trial itself or the analysis of the data. The results of these trials are being submitted to the scrutiny of the world scientific community as soon as they appear.

PERSPECTIVES

Different effector mechanisms involved in the protective immune response against malaria have been suggested (Mazier et al, 1988; Nardin and Nussenzweig, 1993; Druilhe and Pérignon, 1994). Nevertheless, in human populations it is not possible to predict protection based on the traditional approach of the study of antibody or cellular response. SPf66 is an example of this phenomenon, since antibodies induced by vaccination have not correlated with protection (Patarroyo et al, 1988; Beck et al, 1994). Thus, other mechanisms of protection by the vaccine must be postulated. This suggests that an extensive study on the cellular response at a clonal level (Quakyi et al, 1994), preferential induction of Th subsets (Cruz Cubas et al, 1994), antibody-dependent cellular inhibition activity (ADCI) and antibody-dependent cellular cytotoxicity (ADCC), amongst others will need to be considered (Druilhe and Pérignon, 1994).

To overcome the problem of antigenic variation, potentially useful vaccines must protect against the different variants by including either protective sequences common to all variants or protective sequences from each variant. Nevertheless, T cell clones have been reported which have an extensive cross-reactivity with variant sequences (Moreno et al, 1993). These data suggest that polymorphism should not be an insurmountable obstacle in developing subunit vaccines.

Genetic restriction of the immune response to malaria has been observed for both T cell and B cell epitopes (Quakyi et al, 1992; Nardin and Nussenzweig, 1993). A vaccine would have to include multiple T epitopes from different target antigens or alternatively a universal T cell activator epitope. Vaccines based on synthetic peptides must be easily modified to increase their immunogenicity. The modified peptides could be included in a cocktail constructed to benefit the conversion of the host to a 'responder phenotype'.

The problem of the three-dimensional conformation of the peptide in solution should also be addressed. Synthetic peptides and recombinant proteins do not necessarily adopt their native conformation as in the intact molecule, which will consequently affect both the sensitivity and specificity of binding to an antibody or receptor. Although a recent article reports the expression of antigens in their correct conformation (Murphy et al, 1994), this appears to be a rather isolated case, and this particular expression vector merits study. Methods are currently available for conformationally restricting peptides with covalent replacements for hydrogen bonds, thus locking the peptide into a configuration that mimics the epitope's native conformation (Satterthwait et al, 1989, 1990).

Another issue needing to be addressed is poor immunogenicity of deposit-based adjuvants. Several new adjuvants which enhance the uptake and presentation of antigens by antigen-presenting cells and stimulate lymphokine production and modulate T helper and CTL response, are currently being developed (Hui, 1994). However, the limitations of such a new adjuvant formulation would be its side effects and high cost/dose.

Constraints of resources have been the major obstacle in the implementation of a control program for malaria. Local malaria endemicities at the village level show high variability which, makes comparison difficult. Stratification of areas on the basis of the local microepidemiological picture, and rationalizing the use of different control measures within the Public Health Control System are necessary to overcome this problem (Jambulingam et al, 1991).

There is a huge gap in the knowledge that is necessary for the transition from Phase III to Phase IV trials. What is the optimum and minimum information/knowledge required in a given situation to move from controlled trials to routine evaluation of a vaccine? What do we expect from a malaria vaccine in a given eco-epidemiological situation? To what extent will the results of SPf66's trials in The Gambia, Tanzania, Thailand and Latin America correlate/complement each other?

We have already tested the protection of SPf66 under low and high malarial endemicity in Latin America and Tanzania, respectively, two ends of the epidemiological spectrum. The requirements will certainly differ from country to country, considering the different effects, areas, strains, vectors, populations, magnitude of the problem and public health impact. This should lead to an independent, but coordinated approach to assess the potential use of the vaccine in different regions of the world.

An effective malaria vaccine would have tremendous public health and economic consequences. It would reduce childhood mortality in Africa, it would substantially reduce the amount presently spent on treatment, it would improve nutrition and could bring direct economic benefits by reducing absenteeism and by improving work efficiency. In tropical Africa, using a malaria vaccine that costs $10/dose (production by chemical synthesis US$ 0.15 and around US$10 for delivery), avoidance of a clinical attack would cost around $2 and prevention of death, $250/life.

SUMMARY

Although knowledge of the malaria parasite's biology is incomplete, research carried out during the last 40 years has allowed insight into some of the mechanisms the parasite uses to evade host immunity. From this still unclear picture, certain principles have been clarified for the development of a malaria vaccine. One of these is the necessity to adopt an 'antigenic cocktail' approach to synthetic subunit vaccine design. The SPf66 vaccine, developed by our group, is an example of this methodology, which we hope will endorse the success of this approach. Second generation multi-component malaria vaccines should be designed to include a string of epitopes, each of which, when inserted into the preparation in its correct three-dimensional conformation, will elicit a specific host response. Non-specific factors, such as adjuvants and delivery systems, could make a contribution to increase the protective immune response.

Acknowledgment

We dedicate this paper to the people of Colombia. Our work has been supported by the Presidency of Colombia, Ministry of Health of Colombia, the Corporación Andina de Fomento (CAF), Colciencias and the German Leprosy Relief Association (DAHW).

REFERENCES

Aldhous P (1994) Parasitology. Fighting parasites on a shoestring. *Science* **264:** 1857–1859.

Alonso PL, Smith T, Armstrong Schellenberg JRM et al (1994) Randomised trial of efficacy of SPf66 vaccine against *Plasmodium falciparum* malaria in children in southern Tanzania. *Lancet* **344:** 1175–1181.

Amador R, Moreno A, Valero V et al (1992) The first field trials of the chemically synthesized malaria vaccine SPf66: safety, immunogenicity and protectivity. *Vaccine* **10:** 179–184.

Bate CAW & Kwiatkowski D (1994a) Inhibitory immunoglobulin M antibodies to tumor necrosis factor-inducing toxins in patients with malaria. *Infection and Immunity* **62:** 3086–3091.

Bate CAW & Kwiatkowski D (1994b) A monoclonal antibody that recognizes phosphatidylinositol inhibits induction of tumor necrosis factor alpha by different strains of *Plasmodium falciparum*. *Infection and Immunity* **62:** 5261–5266.

Beck H, Felger I, Kabintik S et al (1994) Assessment of the humoral and cell-mediated immunity against the *Plasmodium falciparum* vaccine candidates circumsporozoite protein and Spf66 in adults living in highly endemic malarious areas of Papua New Guinea. *American Journal Tropical Medicine and Hygiene* **51:** 356–364.

Clyde DF (1990) Immunity to falciparum and vivax malaria induced by irradiated sporozoites: a review of the University of Maryland studies. *Bulletin of the WHO* **68:** 9–12.

Collins WE (1992) South American monkeys in the development and testing of malaria vaccines. A review. *Memories Institute Oswaldo Cruz* **87:** 401–406.

Cruz Cubas AB, Gentilini M & Monjour L (1994) Cytokines and T cell response in malaria. *Biomedical Pharmacotherapy* **48:** 27–33.

De La Cruz VF, Maloy WL, Miller LH et al (1989) The immunologic significance of variation within malaria circumsporozoite protein sequences. *Journal of Immunology* **142:** 3568–3575.

Del Giudice G (1991) Towards a malaria vaccine: what is in sight? *Allergologia Et Immunopathologia* **19:** 129–135.

Druilhe P & Pérignon J (1994) Mechanisms of defense against *P. falciparum* asexual blood stages in humans. *Immunology Letters* **41:** 115–120.

Esposito F, Gambella R, Modiano D et al (1991) Waiting for the vaccine: sporozoite vaccine research entails important progress in malaria epidemiology. *Parasitologia* **33:** 85–91.

Good MF (1991) Towards the development of the ideal malaria vaccine. A decade of progress in a difficult field. *Medical Journal of Australia* **154:** 284–289.

Good MF, Saul A & Graves PM (1992) Malaria vaccines. *Biotechnology* **20:** 69–98.

Greenwood BM, Bradley AK, Greenwood AM et al (1987) Mortality and morbidity from malaria among children in a rural area of The Gambia, West Africa. *Transactions of the Royal Society of Tropical Medicine and Hygiene* **81:** 478–486.

Holder AA (1994) Proteins on the surface of the malaria parasite and cell invasion. *Parasitology* **108:** S5-S18.

Hui GSN (1994) Liposomes, muramyl dipeptide derivatives, and nontoxic lipid A derivatives as adjuvants for human malaria vaccines. *American Journal Tropical Medicine and Hygiene* **50:** 41–51.

Jambuligam P, Mohapatra SSS, Govardhini P et al (1991) Microlevel epidemiological variation in malaria and implications on control strategy. *Indian Journal of Medical Research* **93:** 371–378.

Kaslow DC, Quakyi IA & Keister DB (1989) Minimal variation in a vaccine candidate from the sexual stage of *Plasmodium falciparum*. *Molecular and Biochemical Parasitology* **32:** 101–103.

Kolberg R (1994) Parasite control. Finding 'sustainable' ways to prevent parasitic diseases. *Science* **264:** 1859–1861.

Lopez MC, Silva Y, Thomas MC et al (1994) Characterization of SPf(66)n: a chimeric molecule used as a malaria vaccine. *Vaccine* **12:** 585–591.

Lussow AR, Aguado MT, Del Giudice G & Lambert PH (1990) Towards vaccine optimisation. *Immunology Letters* **25:** 255–263.

Marsh K, Otoo L, Hayes RJ et al (1989) Antibodies to blood stage antigens of *Plasmodium falciparum* in rural Gambians and their relation to protection against infection. *Transactions of the Society of Tropical Medicine and Hygiene* **83:** 293–303.

Mazier D, Miltgen F, Nudelman S et al (1988) Pre-erythrocytic stages of plamodia. Role of specific and nonspecific factors. *Cell Biology* **64:** 165–172.

Moreno A, Clavijo P, Edelman R et al (1993) CD4+ T cell clones obtained from *Plasmodium falciparum* sporozoite-immunized volunteers recognize polymorphic sequences of the circumsporozoite protein. *Journal of Immunology* **151:** 489–499.

Murillo LA, Rocha CL, Mora AL et al (1992) Molecular analysis of each HLA DR4 B-1 gene in malaria vaccines. Typing and subtyping by PCR technique and oligonucleotides. *Parasite Immunology* **13:** 201–210.

Murphy VF, Rowan WC, Page MJ & Holder AA (1994) Expression of hybrid malaria antigens in insect cells and their engineering for correct folding and secretion. *Parasitology* **100:** 177–183.

Nardin EH & Nussenzweig RS (1993) T cell responses to pre-erythrocytic stages of malaria: role in protection and vaccine development against pre-erythrocytic stages. *Annual Review of Immunology* **11:** 687–727.

Nussenzweig RS (1990) Recombinant proteins and synthetic peptides as malaria vaccine candidates. *Canadian Journal of Microbiology* **36:** 817–820.

Nussenzweig RS & Long CA (1994) Malaria vaccines: multiple targets. *Science* **265:** 1381–1383.

Nussenzweig RS & Nussenzweig V (1989) Antisporozoite vaccine for malaria: experimental basis and current status. *Reviews of Infectious Diseases* **11 (supplement 3):** 579–585.

Pasloke BL & Howard RJ (1994) The promise of asexual malaria vaccine development. *American Journal of Tropical Medicine and Hygiene* **50:** 3–10.

Patarroyo ME, Romero P, Torres ML et al (1987a) Protective synthetic peptides against experimental *P. falciparum* induced malaria, In Chanock RM, Lerner RA, Brown F & Ginsberg H (eds.) *Vaccines 87* pp 117–124. New York: Cold Spring Harbor Laboratory Press.

Patarroyo ME, Romero P, Torres ML et al (1987b) Induction of protective immunity against experimental infection with malaria using synthetic peptides. *Nature* **328:** 629–632.

Patarroyo ME, Amador R, Clavijo P et al (1988) A synthetic vaccine protects humans against challenge with asexual blood stages of *Plasmodium falciparum* malaria. *Nature* **332:** 158–161.

Patarroyo ME, Vinasco J, Amador R et al (1991) Genetic control of the immune response to a synthetic vaccine against *Plasmodium falciparum*. *Parasite Immunology* **13:** 509–516.

Patarroyo G, Franco L, Amador R et al (1992) Study of the safety and immunogenicity of the synthetic malaria SPf66 vaccine in children aged 1–14 years, *Vaccine* **10:** 175–178.

Quakyi IA, Taylor DW, Johnson AH et al (1992) Development of a malaria T-cell vaccine for blood stage immunity. *Scandinavian Journal of Immunology* **36 (supplement 11):** 9–16.

Quakyi IA, Currier J, Fell A et al (1994) Analysis of human T cell clones specific for conserved peptide sequences within malaria proteins. *Journal of Immunology* **153:** 2082–2092.

Reese R, Trager W, Jensen J et al (1978) Immunization against malaria with antigen from *P. falciparum* cultivated in vitro. *Proceedings of the National Academy of Sciences of the USA* **75:** 5665–5670.

Ringwald P, Peyron F, Lepers JP et al (1993) Parasite virulence factors during falciparum malaria: rosetting, cytoadherence, and modulation of cytoadherence by cytokines. *Infection and Immunity* **61:** 5198–5204.

Rocha CL, Murillo LA, Mora AL et al (1992) Determination of the immunization schedule for field trials with the synthetic malaria vaccine SPf66. *Parasite Immunology* **14:** 95–109.

Rodriguez R, Moreno A, Guzman F et al (1990) Studies in owl monkeys leading to the development of a synthetic vaccine against the asexual blood stages of *Plasmodium falciparum*. *American Journal of Tropical Medicine and Hygiene* **43**: 339–354.

Romero P (1992) Malaria vaccines. *Current Opinion in Cell Biology* **4**: 432–441.

Salcedo M, Barreto L, Rojas M et al (1991) Studies on the humoral immune response to a synthetic vaccine against *Plasmodium falciparum* malaria. *Clinical Experimental Immunology* **84**: 122–128.

Sampértegui F, Estrella B, Moscos J et al (1994) Safety, immunogenicity and protective effect of the SPf66 malaria synthetic vaccine against *Plasmodium falciparum* infection in randomized double-blind placebo-controlled field trials in an endemic area of Ecuador. *Vaccine* **12**: 337–342.

Satterthwait AC, Arrhenius T, Hagopian RA et al (1989) The conformational restriction of synthetic peptides, including a malaria peptide, for use as immunogens. *Philosophical Transactions of the Royal Society of London, Series B* **323**: 3–72.

Satterthwait AC, Chiang LC, Arrhenius T et al (1990) The conformational restriction of synthetic vaccines for malaria. *Bulletin of the World Health Organisation* **68(supplement)**: 17–25.

Shi YP, Alpers MP, Povoa MM & Lal AA (1992) Single amino acid variation in the ookinete vaccine antigen from field isolates of *Plasmodium falciparum*. *Molecular and Biochemical Parasitology* **50**: 179–180.

Special Programme for Research and Training in Tropical Diseases (1988) Role of non-human primates in malaria vaccine development: Memorandum from a WHO Meeting. *Bulletin of the World Health Organization* **66**: 719–728.

Teuscher T, Armstrong Schellenberg JRM, de Azevedo I et al (1994) Spf66, a chemically synthesized subunit malaria vaccine, is safe and immunogenic in Tanzanians exposed to intense malaria transmission. *Vaccine* **12**: 328–336.

Valero MV, Amador R, Galindo C, et al (1993) Vaccination with Spf66, a chemically synthesised vaccine, against *Plasmodium falciparum* malaria in Colombia. *Lancet* **341**: 705–710.

Index